EXCHANGES
FOR ALL
OCCASIONS

EXCHANGES
FOR ALL
OCCASIONS

with Carbohydrate Counting

Pocket Guide to
Healthy Food Choices
Anytime, Anywhere

Marion J. Franz, MS, RD, CDE

IDC Publishing
Minneapolis

IDC Publishing
3800 Park Nicollet Boulevard
Minneapolis, Minnesota 55416-2699
1-888-825-6315
www.idcpublishing.com

ISBN 1-885115-56-3

Printed in the United States of America

Editorial Director/Publisher: Karol Carstensen
Editorial Assistant: Kerri Oachs
Production Manager: Gail Devery
Cover and Text Design: MacLean & Tuminelly

Table of Contents

Introduction

Good nutrition and good health begin with making healthy food choices. Regular physical activity is equally important to good health and contributes to the success of any healthy eating plan. Eating a balanced, healthy diet and staying physically active help you look and feel your best.

While the importance of physical activity to your health and well being can't be stressed enough, this book is about food. Scientists have made great strides in understanding the role of food and nutrition in health and disease, and we now know that healthy food choices not only improve health but can actually help prevent some health problems. Making healthy food choices, along with living an active lifestyle, can reduce your risk of obesity, heart disease, diabetes, high blood pressure, and some forms of cancer.

The purpose of this book is to help you make good food choices in any situation, whether you're enjoying a home-cooked meal, stopping by a fast food restaurant, or celebrating at a New Year's Eve party. It provides comprehensive lists of a variety of foods along with the nutrition information you need to include them in your meals in a healthy way.

Food Exchanges

The exchange lists group foods based on nutritional content. The lists fall into three main groups: carbohydrate, meat and meat substitutes, and fat. Together foods from these groups give us all the nutrients we need to live, grow, and stay healthy.

The Exchange Lists
Carbohydrate Lists
- Starch List
- Fruit List
- Milk List
- Other Carbohydrates List
- Vegetable List

Meat and Meat Substitutes List

Fat List

Free Foods List

Combination Foods List

Of course not all the foods we eat fit neatly into the three main groups. Lasagna, for instance, is made from pasta (starch), beef (meat), cheese (meat substitute), and tomato sauce (vegetable). The Combination Foods List accommodates such foods by giving serving sizes and the exchange values for each. The Free Foods List includes low-calorie, low-fat, low-sugar foods that can be used to round out your meals without worry.

Each list gives food choices and the amount of each food that equals one exchange, or one serving. Each serving from a list is a measured amount of food that has approximately the same carbohydrate, protein, fat, and caloric content as other foods on the same list. Any food on a list can be "exchanged, " or traded, for any other food on the same list *in the amounts given*, because each serving provides the same nutritional value and the same number of calories.

The lists in this book expand on the original exchange list idea by including more food choices in each of the basic exchanges lists and by including exchange lists for different types of foods. The additional lists include more of the kinds of foods that are readily available today such as Indian foods, Mexican foods, Oriental foods, convenience foods and almost anything else you eat or want to eat.

As you think about incorporating healthy eating into your life, remember that food can and does taste good. Enjoy!

CHAPTER 1

Starch List

The Starch List includes a wide variety of foods – breads, cereals, rice, pasta, and other foods made from grains, as well as peas, beans, and lentils. Many of the foods on this list are good choices for you. Like all carbohydrate foods, starches give us energy, and they are often good sources of fiber as well. This list is discussed first because the foods on it are the foundation of a healthy meal plan. Depending on your caloric intake, plan to eat six to eleven starch servings each day.

One starch serving has:
15 grams carbohydrate
3 grams protein
½–1 gram fat
80 calories

One starch serving is:
1 ounce of a bread or snack product
¾ cup dry, unsweetened cereal
½ cup cooked cereal
4–5 snack crackers
½ cup pasta or starchy vegetable
⅓ cup rice, grains, stuffings
1 cup soup
½ cup cooked beans, peas, lentils
3 cups popcorn without added fat

Starch List

Food	Quantity	Carb Choices	Exchanges
Bagel			
Medium (1 oz)	½ bagel	1	1 starch
Large (3.5 oz)	1 bagel	3½	3½ starch
Barley, cooked	⅓ cup	1	1 starch
Beans, baked			
Canned	⅓ cup	1	1 starch
	1 cup	3	3 starch, 1 very lean meat
Canned with franks	½ cup	1	1 starch, 1 high fat meat
Pork and beans	⅓ cup	1	1 starch
Beans, dried, cooked or canned	½ cup	1	1 starch, 1 very lean meat
	1 cup	2	2 starch, 1 very lean meat
Black beans	⅓ cup	1	1 starch
Garbanzo beans	⅓ cup	1	1 starch
Lima beans	½ cup	1	1 starch
Mung beans	⅓ cup	1	1 starch
Navy beans	⅓ cup	1	1 starch
Pinto beans	⅓ cup	1	1 starch
Beans, refried	⅓ cup	1	1 starch, 1 fat
Bean dip, canned	¼ cup	1	1 starch
Biscuit, baking soda or buttermilk	1 (2½" across)	1	1 starch, 1 fat
Black-eyed peas, canned	½ cup	1	1 starch
Bread; *see also* Pocket/Pita bread			
Boston brown bread	1 slice (3" across x ½" thick)	1	1 starch

Food	Quantity	Carb Choices	Exchanges
Corn bread	2" square	1	1 starch, 1 fat
French bread	1 slice (3" thick)	1	1 starch
Home-baked or unsliced bread	1 oz	1	1 starch
Party bread (pumpernickel, rye)	4 slices	1	1 starch
Pumpernickel	1 slice	1	1 starch
Raisin bread, unfrosted	1 slice (1 oz)	1	1 starch
Rye bread	1 slice	1	1 starch
Spoon bread	3½ oz	1	1 starch, 2 fat
Wheat bread	1 slice (1 oz)	1	1 starch
White bread	1 slice (1 oz)	1	1 starch
Bread, reduced calorie	2 slices (1½ oz)	1	1 starch
Bread, tea			
Banana bread	1 slice (1/16 loaf)	1	1 starch, 1 fat
Cranberry bread	1 slice (1½ oz)	1½	1½ starch, 1 fat
Pumpkin bread	1 slice (1½ oz)	1½	1½ starch, 1 fat
Bread crumbs, dry	3 Tbsp	1	1 starch
Breadsticks			
4" long x ½" thick	2 breadsticks	1	1 starch
4" long x ¼" thick	6 breadsticks	1	1 starch
Bulgur, cooked	½ cup	1	1 starch
Bun, hamburger or hot dog	1 bun (2 oz)	2	2 starch
Carob flour	2 Tbsp	1	1 starch
Cereal, ready-to-eat			
All Bran*	½ cup	1	1 starch
All Bran with Extra Fiber*	1 cup	1	1 starch
Apple Raisin Crisp*	⅔ cup	2	2 starch
Bran Buds*	½ cup	1	1 starch
Bran Chex*	½ cup	1	1 starch

Food	Quantity	Carb Choices	Exchanges
Bran Flakes*	⅔ cup	1	1 starch
100% Bran*	½ cup	1	1 starch
Cheerios*	1 cup	1	1 starch
Cheerios*, Apple Cinnamon	½ cup	1	1 starch
Cheerios*, Honey Nut	½ cup	1	1 starch
Corn Bran*	½ cup	1	1 starch
Corn Chex*	¾ cup	1	1 starch
Corn Flakes*	¾ cup	1	1 starch
Crispy Wheaties 'n Raisins*	¾ cup	1½	1½ starch
Fiber One*	⅔ cup	1	1 starch
Fruit and Fibre*	½ cup	1	1 starch
Fruit Muesli*, all varieties	½ cup	2	2 starch
Granola	¼ cup	1	1 starch, 1 fat
Granola, low-fat	¼ cup	1	1 starch
Grape Nuts*	¼ cup	1	1 starch
Grape Nuts* Flakes	¾ cup	1	1 starch
Kix*	1 cup	1	1 starch
Life*	⅔ cup	1	1 starch
Muesli*	¼ cup	1	1 starch
Mueslix* Crispy Blend	⅓ cup	1	1 starch
Mueslix* Golden Crunch	½ cup	1½	1½ starch
Nutri-Grain* Almond Raisin	⅔ cup	2	2 starch
Nutri-Grain* Raisin Bran	⅔ cup	1	1 starch
Nutri-Grain* Wheat	½ cup	1	1 starch
Oat bran	½ cup	1	1 starch
Oatmeal Crisp*	¾ cup	1	1 starch
Puffed Rice*	1½ cups	1	1 starch

Food	Quantity	Carb Choices	Exchanges
Puffed Wheat*	1½ cups	1	1 starch
Raisin Bran*	½ cup	1	1 starch
Raisin Oat Bran*	¾ cup	2	2 starch
Rice Chex*	¾ cup	1	1 starch
Rice Krispies*	¾ cup	1	1 starch
Sunflakes Multi Grain*	¾ cup	1	1 starch
Shredded Wheat*	1 biscuit	1	1 starch
Shredded Wheat Squares*	½ cup	1	1 starch
Special K*	¾ cup	1	1 starch
Sugar-Frosted Flakes*	½ cup	1	1 starch
Team Flakes*	¾ cup	1	1 starch
Total*	¾ cup	1	1 starch
Total* Raisin Bran	1 cup	2	2 starch
Wheat Chex*	½ cup	1	1 starch
Wheaties*	¾ cup	1	1 starch
Cereal, hot			
Cream of Rice*	½ cup	1	1 starch
Cream of Wheat*	½ cup	1	1 starch
Farina	¾ cup	1	1 starch
Malt-O-Meal*	⅔ cup	1	1 starch
Maypo*	½ cup	1	1 starch
Oat bran, cooked	⅓ cup	1	1 starch
Oatmeal, quick or old fashioned	½ cup	1	1 starch
Oatmeal, instant	1 pkt	1	1 starch
Oatmeal, instant flavored	1 pkt	2	2 starch
Ralston*	⅔ cup	1	1 starch
Roman Meal*	½ cup	1	1 starch
Wheatena*	½ cup	1	1 starch
Chapati, 5–6" across	1 chapati	1	1 starch

Food	Quantity	Carb Choices	Exchanges
Cheese sauce (prepared with milk)	½ cup	1	1 starch, 1 high fat meat
Chestnuts	4 large or 6 small	1	1 starch
Corn			
Canned	½ cup	1	1 starch
Cob	1 medium ear	1	1 starch
Cream style	⅓ cup	1	1 starch
Pudding	½ cup	1	1 starch, 1 fat
Cornmeal, dry	3 Tbsp	1	1 starch
Cornstarch	2 Tbsp	1	1 starch
Couscous, cooked	⅓ cup	1	1 starch
Cowpeas, frozen, boiled	½ cup	1	1 starch
Crackers			
Animal crackers	8 crackers	1	1 starch
American Classic°, all varieties	8 crackers	1	1 starch, 1 fat
Cheese-filled crackers	6 (1½ oz)	1½	1½ starch, 2 fat
Cheese Nips°	20 crackers	1	1 starch, 1 fat
Club°	8 crackers	1	1 starch, 1 fat
Goldfish crackers, all varieties	45 crackers	1	1 starch, 1 fat
Graham crackers, 2½" square	3 crackers	1	1 starch
Harvest Crisp°, all varieties	12 crackers	1	1 starch, 1 fat
Matzo, 6" across	1 wafer	1	1 starch
Matzo crackers, 1½" square	7 crackers	1	1 starch
Melba toast, long	4 slices	1	1 starch
Melba toast, rounds	8 crackers	1	1 starch

Food	Quantity	Carb Choices	Exchanges
Oat Bran Krisp®	4 triple crackers	1	1 starch, 1 fat
Oyster crackers	24 large or 42 small	1	1 starch
Peanut-butter filled crackers	6 (1½ oz)	1½	1½ starch, 2 fat
Ritz®, Hi Ho®	6 crackers	1	1 starch, 1 fat
Rusk	2 crackers	1	1 starch
RyKrisp®, all varieties	3 crackers	1	1 starch
Saltines	6 crackers	1	1 starch
Snack Sticks, all varieties	8 crackers	1	1 starch, 1 fat
Sociables®	8 crackers	1	1 starch, 1 fat
Toasted snack crackers, all varieties	8 crackers	1	1 starch, 1 fat
Town House®	8 crackers	1	1 starch, 1½ fat
Triscuit®	6 crackers	1	1 starch, 1 fat
Uneeda® biscuits	5 crackers	1	1 starch, 1 fat
Waverly® wafers	6 crackers	1	1 starch, 1 fat
Wheat Thins®	14 crackers	1	1 starch, 1 fat
Whole wheat crackers	4–6 crackers (1 oz)	1	1 starch, 1 fat
Whole wheat crackers, no fat added	2–5 crackers (¾ oz)	1	1 starch
Zweibach	3 crackers (¾ oz)	1	1 starch
Croissant			
Medium	1 croissant	1½	1½ starch, 2½ fat
Small	1 croissant	1	1 starch, 1½ fat
Croutons	1 cup	1	1 starch
Crumpet	1 crumpet	1	1 starch
English muffin, all varieties	1 muffin	2	2 starch

Food	Quantity	Carb Choices	Exchanges
Falafel, 2" across	3 patties	1	1 starch, 1 med. fat meat, 2 fat
Farfel, dry	3 Tbsp	1	1 starch
Flour	3 Tbsp	1	1 starch
French toast	1 slice	1	1 starch, ½ med. fat meat
Grits, instant, plain or flavored	½ cup or 1 pkt	1	1 starch
Hominy, cooked	½ cup	1	1 starch
Hummus	¼ cup	1	1 starch, 1 fat
Kasha (buckwheat groats)			
Cooked	½ cup	1	1 starch
Puffed	1 cup	1	1 starch
Lentils	½ cup	1	1 starch
Malanga, boiled	⅓ cup	1	1 starch
Marinara sauce	¾ cup	1	1 starch
Millet	¼ cup	1	1 starch
Miso	½ cup	2½	2½ starch, 1 med. fat meat
Muffin mix (as prepared)			
Apple streusel or wild blueberry	1/12 pkg	2	2 starch, 1 fat
Banana	1/12 pkg	1½	1½ starch, 1 fat
Wild blueberry or apple cinnamon, fat-free	1/12 pkg	2	2 starch
Muffins			
Apple cinnamon, banana nut, or blueberry	1 small (1½ oz)	1	1 starch, 1 fat
Carrot nut, chocolate chip, or oatmeal raisin	1 small (1½ oz)	1½	1½ starch, 1 fat

Food	Quantity	Carb Choices	Exchanges
Oat bran or streusel	1 small (1½ oz)	1½	1½ starch, 1½ fat
Muffins, low-fat varieties	1 small (1½ oz)	1	1 starch
Noodles			
Cellophane	¾ cup	1	1 starch
Chinese	⅓ cup	1	1 starch
Chow mein	½ cup	1	1 starch, 1 fat
Ramen	½ pkg (1½ oz)	2	2 starch, 1½ fat
Ramen, low-fat	½ pkg (1½ oz)	3	3 starch
Somen, cooked	⅓ cup	1	1 starch
Spaetzle	⅓ cup	1	1 starch
Udon, cooked	⅓ cup	1	1 starch
Onion rings, frozen	4 rings	1	1 starch, 2 fat
Pancakes, frozen or microwave, 3½" across	2 cakes	1	1 starch, 1 fat
Pancakes (as prepared from mix)	3 cakes (4" across)	2	2 starch, 1 fat
Parsnips, cooked	½ cup	1	1 starch
Pasta, cooked	½ cup	1	1 starch
Patty shell	1 shell	1	1 starch, 3 fat
Peas			
Green, cooked	½ cup	1	1 starch
Split, cooked	½ cup	1	1 starch
Plantain	½ cup	1	1 starch
Pocket/Pita bread			
4½" across	1 pocket/pita	1	1 starch
6½" across	½ pocket/pita	1	1 starch
Poi (taro, cooked)	⅓ cup	1	1 starch
Polenta	⅓ cup	1	1 starch

Food	Quantity	Carb Choices	Exchanges
Popcorn			
Air-popped	5 cups	1	1 starch
Microwave regular	3 cups	1	1 starch, 1 fat
Microwave low-fat or nonfat	3 cups	1	1 starch
Popover	1 small	1	1 starch, 1 fat
Potatoes			
Au gratin, homemade	½ cup	1	1 starch, 2 fat
Au gratin (from mix)	½ cup	1	1 starch, 1 fat
Baked or boiled	1 small (3 oz)	1	1 starch
Baked, with skin	1 medium (7 oz)	3	3 starch
Baked, without skin	1 medium (5½ oz)	2	2 starch
French-fried, frozen	10 strips	1	1 starch, 1 fat
French-fried, restaurant	10 strips	1	1 starch, 2 fat
Hash brown	½ cup	1	1 starch, 2 fat
Mashed	½ cup	1	1 starch
Potatoes O'Brien	½ cup	1	1 starch
Potato pancakes	1 cake	2	2 starch, 2 fat
Potato puffs, frozen	½ cup	1	1 starch, 1 fat
Scalloped	½ cup	1	1 starch, 1 fat
Tater-Tots®	½ cup	1	1 starch, 1 fat
Twice-baked, frozen	½ potato (5 oz)	2	2 starch, 2 fat
Potato chips	12–18 chips (1 oz)	1	1 starch, 2 fat
Fat-free	12–18 chips (1 oz)	1	1½ starch
Potato salad	½ cup	1	1 starch, 2 fat
Potato sticks or shoestrings	¾ cup	1	1 starch, 2 fat
Pretzels	¾ oz	1	1 starch
Mini	12 pretzels	1	1 starch

Food	Quantity	Carb Choices	Exchanges
Very thin twisted	4 pretzels	1	1 starch
Very thin sticks	65 sticks	1	1 starch
Puppodums, plain	2 small	1	1 starch
Quinoa, cooked	⅓ cup	1	1 starch
Rice			
Basmati, cooked	½ cup	1	1 starch
Brown, cooked	⅓ cup	1	1 starch
Fried	⅓ cup	1	1 starch, 1 fat
Instant, cooked	⅓ cup	1	1 starch
Long-grain, cooked	⅓ cup	1	1 starch
White, cooked	⅓ cup	1	1 starch
Wild, cooked	½ cup	1	1 starch
Rice cakes, all flavors, 4" across	2 cakes	1	1 starch
Mini	½ oz	1	1 starch
Rice milk	½ cup	1	1 starch
Roll			
Brown and serve	1 small	1	1 starch
Crescent or twist	1 roll	1	1 starch, 1 fat
Dinner	1 small	1	1 starch
Hard	1 small	1	1 starch
Rutabaga	¾ cup	1	1 starch
Salsify or Oyster Plant	¾ cup	1	1 starch
Scrapple	2 slices (½" thick)	1	1 starch, 1 high fat meat
Snack Foods			
Bugles®, all varieties	30 chips (1 oz)	1	1 starch, 1½ fat
Cheetos®, regular varieties	1 oz	1	1 starch, 2 fat
Cheetos®, light	1 oz	1	1 starch, 1 fat

Food	Quantity	Carb Choices	Exchanges
Chex Snack Mix®, all varieties	⅔ cup (1 oz)	1	1 starch, 1 fat
Fritos® corn chips, all varieties	~34 chips (1 oz)	1	1 starch, 2 fat
Dinosaur Grahams®	1 large	1	1 starch
Doo Dads®	½ cup (1 oz)	1	1 starch, 1 fat
Granola bars, all varieties	1 bar	1½	1½ starch, 1 fat
Party Mix®	¼ cup	1	1 starch, 2 fat
Potato chips	12–18 chips	1	1 starch, 2 fat
Potato chips, fat-free	12–18 chips	1	1½ starch
Power Bar®	1 bar (2 oz)	3	3 starch
Sandwich crackers, cheese or peanut butter filling	3 crackers	1	1 starch, 1 fat
Sesame chips	¼ cup	1	1 starch, 2 fat
Teddy Grahams®	15 crackers	1	1 starch, ½ fat
Soups (prepared with water unless otherwise noted)			
Bean with bacon	1 cup	1½	1½ starch, 1 fat
Bean with ham, chunky	1 cup	2	2 starch, 1 meat
Beef, chunky	1 cup	1	1 starch, 1 meat
Beef noodle	1 cup	1	1 starch
Black bean	1 cup	1	1 starch
Cheese	1 cup	1	1 starch, 2 fat
Chicken, chunky	1 cup	1	1 starch, 1 meat
Chicken noodle	1 cup	1	1 starch
Chicken rice	1 cup	1	1 starch
Chili beef	1 cup	1½	1½ starch, 1 fat
Clam chowder, Manhattan	1 cup	1	1 starch
Clam chowder, New England (prepared with milk)	1 cup	1	1 starch, 1 fat

Food	Quantity	Carb Choices	Exchanges
Cream of asparagus	1 cup	1	1 starch, 1 fat
Cream of mushroom	1 cup	1	1 starch, 1 fat
Cream of potato	1 cup	1	1 starch, 1 fat
Lentil with ham	1 cup	1½	1½ starch, 1 fat
Minestrone	1 cup	1	1 starch
Minestrone, chunky	1 cup	1½	1½ starch
Oyster stew (prepared with milk)	1 cup	1	1 starch, 1 fat
Pea, split, with ham	1 cup	2	2 starch, 1 lean meat
Pea, split, with ham, chunky	1 cup	1½	1½ starch, 1 lean meat
Ramen noodle, all regular varieties	½ pkg	2	2 starch, 1½ fat
Ramen noodle, low-fat	½ pkg	3	3 starch
Tomato	1 cup	1	1 starch
Tomato bisque	1 cup	1½	1½ starch
Tomato rice	1 cup	1½	1½ starch
Turkey, chunky	1 cup	1	1 starch, 1 meat
Turkey noodle	1 cup	1	1 starch
Vegetable, chunky	1 cup	1	1 starch, 1 fat
Vegetable, vegetarian	1 cup	1	1 starch
Vegetable with beef	1 cup	1	1 starch
Won ton soup	1 cup (2 won tons)	½	½ starch
Soybeans, cooked	½ cup	½	½ starch, 1 med. fat meat
Spaghetti sauce	½ cup	1	1 starch
	1 cup	1	1 starch, 1 fat
Squash, winter (acorn, butternut)	1 cup	1	1 starch

Food	Quantity	Carb Choices	Exchanges
Stuffing mix, all varieties, as prepared	⅓ cup	1	1 starch, 1 fat
Succotash	½ cup	1	1 starch
Sweet potato			
Baked	½ medium	1	1 starch
Mashed	⅓ cup	1	1 starch
Taco shell, 6" across	2 shells	1	1 starch, 1 fat
Tapioca, dry	2 Tbsp	1	1 starch
Tempeh	½ cup	1	1 starch, 2 med. fat meat
Tortilla chips	6–12 chips (1 oz)	1	1 starch, 2 fat
Light varieties	6–12 chips (1 oz)	1	1 starch, 1 fat
Baked varieties	9 chips (1 oz)	1½	1½ starch
Tortillas			
Corn, 6" across	1 tortilla	1	1 starch
Flour, 7–8" across	1 tortilla	1	1 starch
Flour, 10" across	1 tortilla	1½	1½ starch
Flour, 12" across	1 tortilla	2	2 starch
Tostada shell	2 shells	1	1 starch, 1 fat
Vegetables, mixed	1 cup	1	1 starch
Waffles, 4½" square	1 waffle	1	1 starch, 1 fat
Mini	4 waffles	1	1 starch, ½ fat
Reduced-fat, 4½" square	1 waffle	1	1 starch
Wheat bran	⅓ cup	1	1 starch
Wheat germ, toasted, plain	¼ cup	1	1 starch, 1 very lean meat
Yam, cooked	½ cup	1	1 starch

CHAPTER 2

Fruit List

Whether fresh, canned, dried, frozen, or as juice, fruits are excellent food choices. They are low in sodium, and they provide important amounts of vitamins A and C and potassium. Fresh fruits are always a good choice; they are satisfying and you can take them anywhere as healthy snacks. Servings of fresh fruits vary in size because of water content. Fruits with a high water content, such as strawberries and watermelon, have a larger portion size than fruits with a low water content, such as bananas and dried fruits.

One fruit serving has:
15 grams of carbohydrate
60 calories

One fruit serving is:
1 small to medium fresh fruit
½ cup canned fruit
¼ cup dried fruit
⅓–½ cup fruit juice

Fruit List

Food	Quantity	Carb Choices	Exchanges
Apple	1 small	1	1 fruit
Dehydrated, dried	4 rings (¼ cup)	1	1 fruit
Apple cider or juice	½ cup	1	1 fruit
Applesauce, unsweetened	½ cup	1	1 fruit
Apricot nectar	⅓ cup	1	1 fruit
Apricots	4 whole (5½ oz)	1	1 fruit
Canned	½ cup	1	1 fruit
Dried	8 halves	1	1 fruit
Asian pear, raw	1 medium	1	1 fruit
Banana	1 small	1	1 fruit
Blackberries	¾ cup	1	1 fruit
Canned in heavy syrup	½ cup	2	2 fruit
Blueberries	¾ cup	1	1 fruit
Canned in heavy syrup	½ cup	2	2 fruit
Wild	½ cup	1	1 fruit
Boysenberries, frozen, unsweetened	1 cup	1	1 fruit
Breadfruit, raw	⅛ medium	1	1 fruit
Cantaloupe	⅓ small	1	1 fruit
Carambala; *see* Star fruit			
Carrot juice	¾ cup (6 oz)	1	1 fruit
Casaba melon	1½ cups cubed	1	1 fruit
Catawba juice	¾ cup	1	1 fruit
Cherimoya, raw	½ medium	1	1 fruit
Cherries			
Sour red, canned, light syrup pack	⅓ cup	1	1 fruit

Food	Quantity	Carb Choices	Exchanges
Sweet, fresh	12 cherries	1	1 fruit
Sweet, canned, juice pack	½ cup	1	1 fruit
Crabapples	¾ cup	1	1 fruit
Cranberry juice cocktail	⅓ cup	1	1 fruit or 1 other carb
Reduced-calorie	1 cup	1	1 fruit or 1 other carb
Cranberry-orange relish	2 Tbsp	1	1 fruit
Currants, red and white, raw	1 cup	1	1 fruit
Dates	3 medium	1	1 fruit
Elderberries	½ cup	1	1 fruit
Feijoa	3 medium	1	1 fruit
Figs	3½ oz	1	1 fruit
Dried	1½ medium	1	1 fruit
Kadota, canned in heavy syrup	½ cup (5 pieces)	2	2 fruit
Fruit cocktail, canned, juice pack	½ cup	1	1 fruit
Fruit juice blends, 100% juice	⅓ cup	1	1 fruit
Fruit spreads			
Kraft® reduced-calorie	8 tsp	1	1 fruit or 1 other carb
Poiret® fruit spread	1 Tbsp	1	1 fruit or 1 other carb
Polaner® All Fruit®	4 tsp	1	1 fruit or 1 other carb
Smucker's®, light	8 tsp	1	1 fruit or 1 other carb

Food	Quantity	Carb Choices	Exchanges
Smucker's®, low sugar	8 tsp	1	1 fruit or 1 other carb
Smucker's® Simply Fruit®	4 tsp	1	1 fruit or 1 other carb
Welch® Totally Fruit®	4 tsp	1	1 fruit or 1 other carb
Gooseberries	1 cup	1	1 fruit
Granadilla; *see* Passion fruit			
Grapefruit	½ fruit	1	1 fruit
Sections, canned	¾ cup	1	1 fruit
Grapefruit juice	½ cup	1	1 fruit
Grape juice	⅓ cup	1	1 fruit
Grapes	17 small	1	1 fruit
Ground-cherries, raw	1 cup	1	1 fruit
Guava	1 medium	1	1 fruit
Canned in heavy syrup	8 pieces	1	1 fruit
Homli fruit	1 medium	1	1 fruit
Honeydew	1 cup cubes	1	1 fruit
Kiwifruit	1 medium	1	1 fruit
Kumquats, raw	5 medium	1	1 fruit
Lemon	3 medium	1	1 fruit
Lemon juice	1 cup	1	1 fruit
Lime	3 medium	1	1 fruit
Lime juice	1 cup	1	1 fruit
Loganberries	¾ cup	1	1 fruit
Loquats	12 fruits	1	1 fruit
Lychees, litchis	½ cup	1	1 fruit
Mandarin oranges			
Canned in light syrup	½ cup	1	1 fruit
Canned in own juice	¾ cup	1	1 fruit

Food	Quantity	Carb Choices	Exchanges
Mango, raw	½ fruit or ½ cup	1	1 fruit
Melon balls, frozen	1 cup	1	1 fruit
Mulberries	1 cup	1	1 fruit
Nectarines	1 small	1	1 fruit
Orange	1 small	1	1 fruit
Orange juice	½ cup	1	1 fruit
Orange-grapefruit juice	½ cup	1	1 fruit
Papaya	½ or 1 cup cubes	1	1 fruit
Papaya nectar	⅓ cup	1	1 fruit
Passion fruit, raw	3 medium	1	1 fruit
Passion fruit juice	½ cup	1	1 fruit
Peach	1 medium or ¾ cup slices	1	1 fruit
Halves, canned, juice pack	2 halves or ½ cup	1	1 fruit
Slices, canned, juice pack	¾ cup	1	1 fruit
Peach nectar	½ cup	1	1 fruit
Pear	½ large (4 oz)	1	1 fruit
Canned, juice pack	2 halves or ½ cup	1	1 fruit
Pear nectar	⅓ cup	1	1 fruit
Persimmons, raw	½ medium	1	1 fruit
Pineapple	¾ cup	1	1 fruit
Canned, juice pack	1½ slices or ½ cup	1	1 fruit
Pineapple juice	½ cup	1	1 fruit
Plums	2 small	1	1 fruit
Canned, juice pack	3 medium or ½ cup	1	1 fruit
Pomegranate, raw	½ medium	1	1 fruit
Prickly pear, raw	1½ medium	1	1 fruit

Food	Quantity	Carb Choices	Exchanges
Pomelo, raw	¾ cup sections	1	1 fruit
Prune juice	⅓ cup	1	1 fruit
Prunes, dried	3 medium	1	1 fruit
Quince, raw	1 medium	1	1 fruit
Raisins	2 Tbsp	1	1 fruit
Raspberries	1 cup	1	1 fruit
Canned in heavy syrup	½ cup	2	2 fruit
Rhubarb, diced	2 cups	1	1 fruit
Sapodilla	1 medium	1	1 fruit
Sapota, raw	1 small	1	1 fruit
Star fruit (carambola)	1½ medium	1	1 fruit
Strawberries	1¼ cups	1	1 fruit
Frozen, unsweetened	1 cup	1	1 fruit
Tamarinds, raw	12 small	1	1 fruit
Tangelos	1 medium	1	1 fruit
Tangerine juice	½ cup	1	1 fruit
Tangerines	2 small	1	1 fruit
Canned, juice pack	⅔ cup	1	1 fruit
Tomato juice	1½ cups	1	1 fruit
Ugli fruit	¾ cup	1	1 fruit
Watermelon	1 slice or 1¼ cup cubes	1	1 fruit

CHAPTER 3

Vegetable List

Meals would be very drab without the color, crispness, and flavor of vegetables. Vegetables are generally low in calories but high in fiber, vitamins, and minerals. Most dark-green and deep-yellow vegetables excel as a source of vitamin A, and many dark-green vegetables also supply valuable amounts of vitamin C. Because of the many nutritional benefits vegetables offer, it is recommended that we eat at least two to three servings each day. Vegetables are listed in the carbohydrate group because they do contain carbohydrate, but in much smaller amounts than starches, fruits, or milk.

One vegetable serving has:
5 grams carbohydrate
2 grams protein
20–25 calories

One vegetable serving is:
½ cup cooked vegetables
½ cup vegetable juice
1 cup raw vegetables

Vegetable List

Food	Quantity	Exchanges
Artichoke		
Base and soft end of leaves, cooked	½ medium	1 veg
Heart, cooked	½ heart	1 veg
Jerusalem artichokes	¼ cup	1 veg
Asparagus	7 spears	1 veg
Bamboo shoots, cooked	½ cup	1 veg
Beets, cooked	½ cup	1 veg
Bell pepper	1 medium	1 veg
Bok choy (Chinese chard), canned	1 cup	1 veg
Borscht	½ cup	1 veg
Broccoli, cooked	½ cup	1 veg
Brussels sprouts	3 sprouts	1 veg
Cabbage, boiled	½ cup	1 veg
Cactus leaves, Napoles	1 medium leaf	1 veg
Carrot	1 large	1 veg
Carrot juice	¼ cup	1 veg
Cauliflower	⅙ medium head	1 veg
Celery	2 medium stalks	1 veg
Chayote, cooked	½ medium or ½ cup	1 veg
Chinese cabbage, Nappa, raw	2 cups shredded	1 veg
Collards, boiled	½ cup	1 veg
Cucumber	⅓ medium	1 veg
Daikon, raw	1 cup	1 veg
Dandelion greens, cooked	½ cup	1 veg
Eggplant, cooked	1 cup cubes	1 veg

Food	Quantity	Exchanges
Green beans	½ cup	1 veg
Heart of palm	½ cup or 3 sticks	1 veg
Italian green beans	½ cup	1 veg
Jicama, raw	½ cup	1 veg
Kale, cooked	½ cup	1 veg
Kohlrabi, raw or cooked	½ cup	1 veg
Leeks, raw	½ cup	1 veg
Lettuce		
Iceberg	⅙ large head	1 veg
Leaf	3 cups shredded	1 veg
Mushrooms	8 medium	1 veg
Mustard greens, cooked	1 cup	1 veg
Okra, cooked	½ cup	1 veg
Onions, cooked	½ cup	1 veg
Pea pods, cooked	½ cup	1 veg
Pumpkin, mashed	½ cup	1 veg
Radishes	5 medium	1 veg
Rhubarb	1 cup	1 veg
Rutabaga, cooked	½ cup	1 veg
Salsa dip	¼ cup	1 veg
Sauerkraut, canned	½ cup	1 veg
Snap beans, cooked	½ cup	1 veg
Snow peas, cooked	½ cup	1 veg
Spinach	1 cup raw or ½ cup cooked	1 veg
Creamed	½ cup	1 veg, 1 fat
Sprouts (alfalfa, bean, soybean)	1 cup raw or ¾ cup cooked	1 veg
Summer squash, cooked	½ cup	1 veg
Tomatillos	2 medium	1 veg

Food	Quantity	Exchanges
Tomato juice	½ cup	1 veg
Tomato	1 whole	1 veg
Paste	2 Tbsp	1 veg
Puree	¼ cup	1 veg
Sauce	⅓ cup	1 veg
Stewed	½ cup	1 veg
Turnip greens, cooked	½ cup	1 veg
Vegetable juice cocktail	½ cup	1 veg
Water chestnuts, canned	6 whole	1 veg
Wax beans	½ cup	1 veg
White mustard cabbage, cooked	½ cup	1 veg
Yard-long beans, cooked	4 pods	1 veg
Zucchini	1 medium	1 veg

CHAPTER 4

Milk List

The Milk List is relatively short but packed with good food choices. Milk and milk products give our bodies calcium, which helps build strong bones and teeth, and protein, which helps repair tissues. Milk and milk products such as yogurt also contain about twelve to fifteen grams of carbohydrate per serving. It's important to eat two to three servings from this list each day – two for most people and three for women who are pregnant or breastfeeding. Teenagers and young adults to age twenty-four need three servings as well.

One milk serving has:
12 grams carbohydrate
8 grams protein
trace amounts of fat
90 calories

One milk serving is:
1 cup skim or 1% milk
8 ounces plain, nonfat yogurt
½ cup evaporated skim milk

Milk List

Food	Quantity	Carb Choices	Exchanges
Alba® cocoa mix, powder	~19 gm pkt	1	1 milk
Alba® Fit 'n Frosty®	~21 gm pkt	1	1 milk
Buttermilk, nonfat or low-fat	1 cup	1	1 milk
Chocolate milk, 1%	1 cup	1	1 milk
Cocoa/hot chocolate; *see* Other Carbohydrates List			
Evaporated milk			
Skim, canned	½ cup	1	1 milk
Whole, canned	½ cup	1	1 milk, 1 ½ fat
Filled milk	1 cup	1	1 milk, 1 fat
Goat's milk	1 cup	1	1 milk, 1 ½ fat
Instant breakfast; *see* Other Carbohydrates List			
Kefir	1 cup	1	1 milk, 1 ½ fat
Lactaid®	1 cup	1	1 milk
Milk			
Skim milk	1 cup	1	1 milk
½% milk	1 cup	1	1 milk
1% milk	1 cup	1	1 milk, ½ fat
2% milk	1 cup	1	1 milk, 1 fat
Whole milk	1 cup	1	1 milk, 2 fat
Milk, nonfat dry	¼ cup dry mix	1	1 milk
Rice Dream®	1 cup	2	2 other carb
Soy milk	1 cup	1 ½	1 ½ milk, 1 fat
Light	1 cup	1	1 milk
Sweet acidophilus	1 cup	1	1 milk, 1 fat
Weight Watchers® shake mixes	1 envelope	1	1 milk

Food	Quantity	Carb Choices	Exchanges
Yogurt			
Custard style, plain	1 cup (8 oz)	1½	1½ milk, 1 fat
Custard style, flavored	¾ cup (6 oz)	2	2 milk, 1 fat
Fruit-flavored	1 cup (8 oz)	3	1 milk, 2 other carb
Fruit-flavored, light	¾ cup (6 oz)	1	1 milk
Fruit-flavored, nonfat or low-fat with sugar substitute	1 cup (8 oz)	1	1 milk
Plain, low-fat	¾ cup (6 oz)	1	1 milk, 1 fat
Plain, nonfat	¾ cup (6 oz)	1	1 milk

CHAPTER 5

Other Carbohydrates List

"**O**ther carbohydrates" are foods with appealing tastes but not much to offer nutritionally – foods like cakes, pies, cookies, jam, candy, and other sweets with added sugar. Typically high in fat and added sugars, these foods give us empty calories with no important vitamins and minerals. Substitute "other carbohydrates" for starch, fruit, or milk exchanges (and fats, if necessary). Watch portion sizes carefully; they are often small.

One serving has:
15 grams carbohydrate
Varying amounts of protein, fat, and calories

One serving is:
1 unfrosted cake or brownie, 2" square
1 cookie, 3" across
2 small cookies
½ cup ice cream
½ cup frozen yogurt

Other Carbohydrates List

Food	Quantity	Carb Choices	Exchanges
Bread pudding	½ cup	2½	2½ other carb, 1½ fat
Brownie, unfrosted	2" square	1	1 other carb, 1 fat
Cake			
Frosted	2" square	2	2 other carb, 1 fat
Unfrosted	2" square	1	1 other carb, 1 fat
Cake (as prepared from mix)			
Angel food cake, unfrosted	¹⁄₁₂ cake	2	2 other carb
Applesauce spice cake, unfrosted	¹⁄₁₂ cake	2	2 other carb, 2 fat
Banana cake, unfrosted	¹⁄₁₂ cake	2	2 other carb, 2 fat
Carrot cake, unfrosted	¹⁄₁₂ cake	2	2 other carb, 1 fat
Gingerbread cake, unfrosted	¹⁄₁₂ cake	2	2 other carb, 1 fat
Candies, hard	3 average	1	1 other carb
Chocolate milk, low-fat	1 cup	2	2 other carb, 1 fat
Chocolate syrup	2 Tbsp	1	1 other carb
Chocolate wafers	3 wafers	1	1 other carb
Cocoa/hot chocolate mix	3 Tbsp	1½	1½ other carb
Fat-free	3 Tbsp	½	½ other carb
No sugar added, reduced calorie	3 Tbsp	1	1 other carb

Food	Quantity	Carb Choices	Exchanges
Cookies			
1¾" across	2 cookies	1	1 other carb, 1 fat
3" across	1 cookie	1	1 other carb, 1 fat
Animal crackers	8 cookies	1	1 other carb
Dinosaur cookies, mini	14 cookies	1	1 other carb, ½ fat
Fig Newtons® or fig bars	2 cookies	1½	1½ other carb
Fortune cookies	2 cookies	1	1 other carb
Frookies®	2 cookies	1	1 other carb, 1 fat
Gingersnaps	3 cookies	1	1 other carb
Ladyfingers®	2 cookies	1	1 other carb
Lorna Doone® shortbread	4 cookies	1	1 other carb, 1 fat
Nilla® vanilla wafers	4 cookies	1	1 other carb, ½ fat
Oreo® sandwich cookies	2 cookies	1	1 other carb, 1 fat
Sandwich cookie with creme filling	2 small	1	1 other carb, 1 fat
Sugar wafers	2 cookies	1	1 other carb, 1 fat
Vanilla wafers	8 cookies	1½	1½ other carb, 1 fat
Cookies, fat-free	2 small	1	1 other carb
Corn syrup or honey	1 Tbsp	1	1 other carb
Cranberry sauce	¼ cup	2	2 other carb
Cream puff shell	1 small	1	1 other carb, 2 fat

Food	Quantity	Carb Choices	Exchanges
Cupcake, frosted	1 small	2	2 other carb, 1 fat
Custard, baked	½ cup	1	1 other carb, 1 med. fat meat
Danish	1 medium	2½	2½ other carb, 2 fat
Doughnut			
Glazed, 3¾" across	1 doughnut	2	2 other carb, 2 fat
Plain cake	1 medium	1½	1½ other carb, 2 fat
Eggnog, nonalcoholic	½ cup	1	1 other carb, 2 fat
Frozen yogurt			
Fat-free, no sugar added	½ cup	1	1 other carb
Low-fat or fat-free	⅓ cup	1	1 other carb
Fruit and cream bar, frozen	1 bar	1	1 other carb
Fruit ice	¼ cup	1	1 other carb
Fruit juice bar, 100% juice	1 bar	1	1 other carb
Fruit Roll-Ups®	1 (½ oz)	1	1 other carb
Fruit snacks, chewy	1 roll (¾ oz)	1	1 other carb
Fruit spreads	1 Tbsp	1	1 other carb
Gatorade®	1 cup	1	1 other carb
Gelatin, regular	½ cup	1	1 other carb
Gelatin desserts	½ cup	1	1 other carb
Granola bars	1 bar	1	1 other carb, 1 fat
Fat-free	1 bar	2	2 other carb
Gumdrops	18 average	1	1 other carb
Hawaiian Punch®, reduced-calorie	1 cup	1	1 other carb

Food	Quantity	Carb Choices	Exchanges
Honey	1 Tbsp	1	1 other carb
Ice cream, all flavors	½ cup	1	1 other carb, 2 fat
Fat-free, no sugar added	½ cup	1	1 other carb
Light	½ cup	1	1 other carb, 1 fat
Ice cream bar	1 bar	1	1 other carb, 2 fat
No sugar added	1 bar	1	1 other carb, 2 fat
Ice cream sandwich	1 sandwich	2	2 other carb, 1 fat
No sugar added	1 sandwich	1½	1½ other carb, 1 fat
Instant Breakfast®, fat-free			
Mix only	1 pkg dry	2	2 other carb
Prepared with skim milk	1 pkg + 1 cup milk	2	1 milk, 1 other carb
Instant Breakfast®, fat-free no sugar added			
Mix only	1 pkg dry	1	1 other carb
Prepared with skim milk	1 pkg + 1 cup milk	2	1 milk, 1 other carb
Jam or jelly, regular	1 Tbsp	1	1 other carb
Jelly beans	9 candies	1	1 other carb
Lemon drops	8 candies	1	1 other carb
Lemonade, punch, or fruit drink	½ cup	1	1 other carb
LifeSavers®	8 candies	1	1 other carb
Marshmallows	3 large	1	1 other carb

Food	Quantity	Carb Choices	Exchanges
Pie			
Fruit with 2 crusts	⅙ pie	3	2 other carb, 1 fruit, 2 fat
Pumpkin or custard	⅛ pie	1	1 other carb, 2 fat
Pie crust	⅙ crust	1	1 other carb, 2 fat
Pound cake, unfrosted	½" slice	1½	1½ other carb, 1 fat
Pudding (all flavors)			
Regular (prepared with skim milk)	½ cup	2	2 other carb, 1 fat
Sugar-free (prepared with skim milk)	½ cup	1	1 other carb
Pudding pops, frozen	1 pop	1	1 other carb
Rice pudding	½ cup	2	2 other carb, 1 fat
Salad dressing, fat-free	¼ cup	1	1 other carb
Sherbet	¼ cup	1	1 other carb
Shortcake, 3" across	1 cake	1	1 other carb
Snapple® beverage	¾ cup (6 oz)	1	1 other carb
Snap-Up® beverage	¾ cup (6 oz)	1	1 other carb
Soft drinks (soda pop), regular	¾ cup (6 oz)	1	1 other carb
Sorbet	¼ cup	1	1 other carb
Sugar, granulated	4 tsp	1	1 other carb
Sundance® sparkling mineral water, juice added	5 oz	1	1 other carb
Sweet roll	1 (2½ oz)	2½	2½ other carb, 2 fat

Food	Quantity	Carb Choices	Exchanges
Syrup, maple	1 Tbsp	1	1 other carb
	¼ cup	4	4 other carb
Light	2 Tbsp	1	1 other carb
Tapioca pudding	½ cup	2	2 other carb, 1 fat
Tropicana® sparkling mineral water, juice added	5 oz	1	1 other carb
Yogurt, low-fat fruited	1 cup	3	2 other carb, 1 milk

CHAPTER 6

Meat and Meat Substitutes List

Foods on the Meat and Meat Substitutes List are impor-tant sources of protein, which helps our bodies form new tissue, repair damaged tissue, and maintain healthy skin, muscles, and blood. Meat and meat substitutes include red meat, poultry, and fish, as well as other foods that are nutritionally similar to meats – cheese, eggs, nuts, and dried peas, beans, and lentils. Beans, peas, and lentils are on both the starch and meat lists because they contain both carbohydrate and a significant amount of protein. Most people need about two to three small servings of meat or meat substitute daily, or about six ounces (six exchanges).

One medium fat meat serving has:
7 grams protein
5 grams fat
75 calories

One medium fat meat serving is:
1 ounce pot roast or
    ground beef
1 ounce string cheese
1 ounce pork chop
1 ounce cheese or processed
    meat with 4–6 grams
    of fat

Meat List

Food	Quantity	Exchanges
Bacon (20 slices/lb)	3 slices	1 high fat meat
Beans, dried, cooked	½ cup	1 starch, 1 very lean meat
	1 cup	2 starch, 1 lean meat
Beef		
Barbecue ribs	1 oz	1 high fat meat
Beef breakfast strips	2 slices (1 oz)	1 high fat meat
Beef jerky	½ oz	1 very lean meat
Blade steak or pot roast	1 oz	1 med. fat meat
Brisket	1 oz	1 high fat meat
Brisket, lean	1 oz	1 med. fat meat
Chipped beef	1 oz	1 very lean meat
Chuck, arm pot roast	1 oz	1 lean meat
Chuck steak or roast	1 oz	1 med. fat meat
Club steak	1 oz	1 med. fat meat
Corned beef	1 oz	1 med. fat meat
Corned beef brisket	1 oz	1 high fat meat
Cubed steak	1 oz	1 lean meat
Eye of round, USDA Select or Choice grade, roast and steak	1 oz	1 lean meat
Family steak	1 oz	1 lean meat
Filet mignon	1 oz	1 lean meat
Flank steak, USDA Select or Choice grade	1 oz	1 lean meat
Ground beef	1 oz	1 med. fat meat
Ground beef, drained	½ cup	3 med. fat meat

Food	Quantity	Exchanges
Ground round or sirloin, very lean (90% lean)	1 oz	1 lean meat
Hamburger, more than 20% fat	1 oz	1 high fat meat
Kabob cubes	1 oz	1 lean meat
Loin strip steaks	1 oz	1 lean meat
Meatballs	1 oz	1 med. fat meat
Meatloaf	1 oz	1 med. fat meat
New York strip steak	1 oz	1 med. fat meat
Porterhouse steak, trimmed of fat	1 oz	1 med. fat meat
Porterhouse steak, USDA Select or Choice grade	1 oz	1 lean meat
Prime rib or steak, untrimmed	1 oz	1 high fat meat
Prime rib, trimmed of fat	1 oz	1 med. fat meat
Rib roast	1 oz	1 med. fat meat
Rib roast, USDA Select or Choice grade	1 oz	1 lean meat
Roast beef, thin sliced	1 oz	1 very lean meat
Round bottom roast, USDA Select or Choice grade	1 oz	1 lean meat
Round tip roast and steak	1 oz	1 lean meat
Round top or London Broil steaks	1 oz	1 lean meat
Rump roast, USDA Select or Choice grade	1 oz	1 lean meat
Scallopini	1 oz	1 lean meat
Shank	1 oz	1 lean meat
Short ribs	1 oz	1 med. fat meat
Shoulder roast	1 oz	1 med. fat meat

Food	Quantity	Exchanges
Sirloin tip roast	1 oz	1 med. fat meat
Sirloin top steak, USDA Select or Choice grade	1 oz	1 lean meat
Skirt steak	1 oz	1 lean meat
Stew meat	1 oz	1 lean meat
Sweetbreads	1 oz	1 lean meat
T-bone steak	1 oz	1 med. fat meat
T-bone, USDA Select or Choice grade	1 oz	1 lean meat
Tenderloin steak	1 oz	1 lean meat
Tenderloin tips	1 oz	1 lean meat
Tenderloin, USDA Select or Choice grade	1 oz	1 lean meat
Tongue	1 oz	1 med. fat meat
Beefalo	1 oz	1 very lean meat
Beerwurst	1 oz	1 high fat meat
Bratwurst	1 link	2 high fat meat, 1 fat
Braunschweiger	1 oz	1 high fat meat
Buffalo	1 oz	1 very lean meat
Capon	1 oz	1 lean meat
Caviar, black and red	2 Tbsp	1 med. fat meat
Cheese		
American cheese or American cheese food	1 oz	1 high fat meat
Blue cheese	1 oz	1 high fat meat
Borden® Lite-Line® cheeses	1 oz	1 lean meat
Cheese ball or log	1 oz	1 high fat meat
Cheese spread	2 Tb	1 high fat meat
Cold pack cheese food	1 oz	1 high fat meat

Food	Quantity	Exchanges
Cottage cheese, nonfat or low-fat	¼ cup	1 very lean meat
Cottage cheese, 4.5% fat	¼ cup	1 lean meat
Crystal Farm® light and reduced-fat cheeses	1 oz	1 lean meat
Fat Free, Most types	1 oz	1 very lean meat
Feta	1 oz	1 med. fat meat
Healthy Choice® fat-free cheese	1 oz	1 very lean meat
Kaukauna® Lite cheese product	1 oz	1 lean meat
Kraft® fat-free cheese	1 oz	1 very lean meat
Kraft® flavored spreads	1 oz	1 med. fat meat
Kraft light and low-fat singles	1 oz	1 lean meat
Kraft® Light 'n Lively®	1 oz	1 lean meat
Laughing Cow® low-fat	1 oz	1 lean meat
Lifetime® low-fat	1 oz	1 lean meat
Light Philadelphia® cream cheese	1 oz	1 med. fat meat
Light 'n Lively® varieties	1 oz	1 med. fat meat
Mozzarella, natural (part skim)	1 oz	1 med. fat meat
Mozzarella, whole milk	1 oz	1 high fat meat
Parmesan, grated	2 Tbsp	1 lean meat
Parmesan, hard	½ oz	1 med. fat meat
Regular, most tupes	1 oz	1 high fat meat
Ricotta, low-fat	2 Tbsp (1 oz)	1 lean meat
Ricotta, natural	¼ cup (2 oz)	1 med. fat meat
Ricotta, whole milk	1 oz	1 high fat meat
Romano	½ oz	1 med. fat meat

Food	Quantity	Exchanges
Sargento® light string cheese	1 oz	1 lean meat
Sargento® pot cheese	1½ oz	1 lean meat
String cheese	1 oz	1 med. fat meat
Weight Watchers® low-fat cheese slices	1 oz	1 lean meat
Weight Watchers® cream cheese spread	1 oz	1 lean meat
Weight Watchers® natural cheddar	1 oz	1 med. fat meat
Chicken		
Breaded and fried	3 oz	1 starch, 3 med. fat meat, 1–2 fat
Canned	1 oz	1 lean meat
Chicken spread	2 Tbsp (1 oz)	1 med. fat meat
Dark meat, no skin	1 oz	1 lean meat
Dark meat, with skin	1 oz	1 med. fat meat
Diced chicken	¼ cup	1 very lean meat
Fried with skin	1 oz	1 med. fat meat
Giblets or gizzard	1 oz	1 lean meat
Ground chicken	1 oz	1 med. fat meat
Livers, simmered	4 average	1 lean meat
Nuggets	3 oz	1 starch, 2 med. fat meat, 1 fat
Patties, breaded, fried	3 oz	1 starch, 2 med. fat meat, 1 fat
Southern fried chicken	3 oz	1 starch, 2 med. fat meat, 2 fat
White meat, no skin	1 oz	1 very lean meat
White meat, with skin	1 oz	1 lean meat
Chitterlings	1 oz	1 high fat meat

Food	Quantity	Exchanges
Clams	4 small	1 very lean meat
Cocktail wieners	3 wieners	1 high fat meat
Cold cuts		
Barbecue loaf, pork and beef	2 slices (1 oz)	1 med. fat meat
Boiled ham	2 slices	1 lean meat
Bologna	1 oz	1 high fat meat
Corned beef loaf, jellied	1 oz	1 lean meat
Deli thin, shaved meats	1 oz	1 very lean meat
Ham and cheese loaf	1 oz	1 med. fat meat
Headcheese	1 oz	1 med. fat meat
Old-fashioned loaf	1 oz	1 med. fat meat
Olive loaf	1 oz	1 high fat meat
Pastrami	1 oz	1 high fat meat
Pickle & pimiento loaf	1 oz	1 high fat meat
Salami	1 oz	1 high fat meat
Summer sausage (thuringer)	1 oz	1 high fat meat
Turkey cotto salami	1 oz	1 med. fat meat
Turkey pastrami (3 grams or less fat per ounce)	1 oz	1 lean meat
Turkey summer sausage (3 grams or less fat per ounce)	1 oz	1 med. fat meat
Cold cuts, low-fat	2 slices	1 lean meat
Cornish hen, no skin	1 oz	1 very lean meat
Crab		
Blue and king, steamed	1 oz	1 very lean meat
Canned meat	¼ cup	2 very lean meat
Crab cakes	1 medium	2 lean meat
Crab Dungeness	1 oz	1 very lean meat

Food	Quantity	Exchanges
Crayfish	16 crayfish	1 very lean meat
Duck, well-drained of fat, no skin	1 oz	1 lean meat
Eggs	1 egg	1 med. fat meat
Egg omelet	2 eggs	2 med. fat meat, 1 fat
Egg substitutes, plain	¼ cup	1 very lean meat
Egg whites	2 egg whites	1 very lean meat
Falafel, 2" across	3 patties (2 oz)	1 starch, 1 med. fat meat, 2 fat
Fish		
Anchovy, drained	7 anchovies	1 med. fat meat
Baked or broiled fish, most types	1 oz	1 very lean meat
Catfish, baked or broiled	1 oz	1 lean meat
Cod, baked or broiled	1 oz	1 very lean meat
Fish sticks	4 sticks	1 starch, 1 med. fat meat
Fried fish	1 oz	1 med. fat meat
Herring, uncreamed or smoked	1 oz	1 lean meat
Mackerel, baked or broiled	1 oz	1 med. fat meat
Salmon (Atlantic or coho)	1 oz	1 lean meat
Salmon, pink, canned in water	1 oz	1 very lean meat
Salmon, red, canned	1 oz	1 lean meat
Tuna, canned in oil, drained	1 oz	1 lean meat
Tuna, canned in water	1 oz	1 very lean meat

Food	Quantity	Exchanges
Franks		
Regular (beef or pork, 10/lb)	1 frank	1 high fat meat, 1 fat
Light (chicken, turkey, beef, or pork, 10/lb)	1 frank	1 high fat meat
Fat-free (10/lb)	1 frank	1 very lean meat
Frog legs	3 medium	1 very lean meat
Goose, well-drained of fat, no skin	1 oz	1 lean meat
Ham salad or spread	2 Tbsp (1 oz)	1 med. fat meat
Ham		
Boneless smoked	1 oz	1 lean meat
Canned or cured	1 oz	1 lean meat
Country style	1 oz	1 high fat meat
Fresh	1 oz	1 lean meat
Minced	1 oz	1 med. fat meat
Hot dogs; *see* Franks		
Knockwurst	1 oz	1 high fat meat
Lamb		
Chops, sirloin or small loin	1 oz	1 lean meat
Cubes, stew	1 oz	1 lean meat
Ground	1 oz	1 med. fat meat
Leg of lamb, whole or boneless	1 oz	1 lean meat
Loin roast	1 oz	1 lean meat
Rib roast	1 oz	1 med. fat meat
Shish kebob	1 oz	1 lean meat
Shoulder roast	1 oz	1 lean meat
Sirloin roast	1 oz	1 lean meat

Food	Quantity	Exchanges
Lentils, dried, cooked	½ cup	1 starch, 1 very lean meat
Liver (high in cholesterol)	1 oz	1 lean meat
Liverwurst	1 oz	1 high fat meat
Lobster	1 oz	1 very lean meat
Miso	½ cup	2½ starch, 1 med. fat meat
Mussels	1 oz	1 very lean meat
Nuts		
Almonds	24 (1 oz)	1 med. fat meat, 2 fat
Cashews	18 (1 oz)	1 med. fat meat, 2 fat
Filberts (hazelnuts)	12 (1 oz)	1 med. fat meat, 2 fat
Mixed nuts, dry or oil roasted	¼ cup (1 oz)	1 med. fat meat, 2 fat
Peanuts	¼ cup (1 oz)	1 med. fat meat, 2 fat
Pistachios	47 (1 oz)	1 med. fat meat, 2 fat
Nut butters		
Almond butter or almond paste	1 Tbsp	1 high fat meat or 2 fat
Peanut butter, creamy or chunky	1 Tbsp	1 high fat meat
	2 Tbsp	1 high fat meat, 1 fat
Sesame butter (tahini)	1 Tbsp	1 high fat meat
Octopus	1 oz	1 very lean meat
Ostrich	1 oz	1 very lean meat

Food	Quantity	Exchanges
Oysters, steamed	6 medium	1 lean meat
Oysters, breaded and fried	3 oz	1 starch, 1 med. fat meat, 1 fat
Pâte, chicken liver	1 oz	1 med. fat meat
Peas, dried, cooked	½ cup	1 starch, 1 very lean meat
Pepperoni	1 oz	1 high fat meat
Pheasant, no skin	1 oz	1 very lean meat
Pig's feet, cured, pickled	1 oz	1 high fat meat
Pork; *see also* Bacon; Chitterlings; Ham		
Arm, picnic, roasted or cured	1 oz	1 med. fat meat
Barbecue ribs	1 oz	1 high fat meat
Boston butt	1 oz	1 med. fat meat
Breakfast strips	2 slices	1 high fat meat
Canadian-style bacon	1 oz	1 lean meat
Center loin chop	1 oz	1 lean meat
Chop	1 oz	1 med. fat meat
Country ribs	1 oz	1 high fat meat
Cutlet	1 oz	1 med. fat meat
Ground pork	1 oz	1 high fat meat
Headcheese	1 oz	1 med. fat meat
Loin blade	1 oz	1 med. fat meat
Loin roast, boneless	1 oz	1 lean meat
Rib chop	1 oz	1 lean meat
Rib roast, boneless	1 oz	1 lean meat
Rump, roasted	1 oz	1 med. fat meat
Shank, roasted	1 oz	1 med. fat meat
Shoulder, roasted	1 oz	1 med. fat meat
Sirloin chop, boneless	1 oz	1 lean meat

Food	Quantity	Exchanges
Sirloin roast	1 oz	1 lean meat
Spareribs	1 oz	1 high fat meat
Tenderloin	1 oz	1 lean meat
Top loin chop, boneless	1 oz	1 lean meat
Quail	1 oz	1 very lean meat
Rabbit	1 oz	1 lean meat
Sausage		
Blood sausage (blood pudding)	1 oz	1 high fat meat
Chorizo	1 link	2 high fat meat, 1 fat
Kielbasa (with 3 grams or less fat per ounce)	1 oz	1 lean meat
Liver sausage	1 oz	1 high fat meat
Polish sausage	1 oz	1 high fat meat
Pork sausage, cooked	2 links or 1 patty	1 high fat meat
Smoked link sausage	1 link	1 high fat meat
Vienna sausage, regular	4 links (2 oz)	1 high fat meat, 1 fat
Vienna sausage (with 1 gram or less fat per ounce)	1 oz	1 very lean meat
Vienna sausage (with approximately 5 grams of fat per ounce)	1 oz	1 med. fat meat
Scallops, broiled	2 large or 5 small	1 very lean meat
Scrapple	1 slice (½" thick)	½ starch, ½ high fat meat
Seafood or shellfish, imitation	1 oz	1 very lean meat

Food	Quantity	Exchanges
Seeds		
Pumpkin or squash	¼ cup (1 oz)	1 med. fat meat, 2 fat
Sunflower	¼ cup (1 oz)	1 med. fat meat, 2 fat
Watermelon seeds	95 (1 oz)	1 med. fat meat, 2 fat
Shrimp		
Boiled	1 oz	1 very lean meat
Breaded, fried	12 shrimp (4 oz)	1 starch, 3 med. fat meat
Soy milk	1 cup	1½ starch, 1 med. fat meat
Soy protein, textured	1 cup	1 starch, 3 very lean meat
Soynuts	½ oz	1 lean meat
Spam*	1 oz	1 high fat meat
Squab (pigeon)	1 oz	1 lean meat
Squid	1 oz	1 very lean meat
Squirrel, roasted	1 oz	1 very lean meat
Tempeh	¼ cup	1 med. fat meat
Tofu	½ cup (2¼" block)	1 med. fat meat
Turkey		
Dark meat, no skin	1 oz	1 lean meat
Ground turkey	1 oz	1 med. fat meat
Smoked breast	1 oz	1 very lean meat
Turkey ham (with 1 gram or less fat per ounce)	1 oz	1 very lean meat
White meat, no skin	1 oz	1 very lean meat

Food	Quantity	Exchanges
Veal		
Chop, loin or sirloin	1 oz	1 lean meat
Cubes for kabobs	1 oz	1 lean meat
Cutlet	1 oz	1 lean meat
Cutlet, ground or cubed, unbreaded	1 oz	1 med. fat meat
Roast	1 oz	1 lean meat
Scallopine	1 oz	1 lean meat
Steak cutlet	1 oz	1 lean meat
Stew cubes	1 oz	1 lean meat
Venison	1 oz	1 very lean meat

Wieners; *see* Cocktail wieners; Franks

CHAPTER 7

Fat List

The Fat List is divided into three types of fat: saturated fat, monounsaturated fat, and polyunsaturated fat. Saturated fats are associated with high blood cholesterol levels, and a diet high in saturated fat can raise your risk of heart disease and cancer. Monounsaturated fats can lower the body's level of harmful LDL-cholesterol while preserving HDL-cholesterol, which helps protect against heart disease. Choose most of your fat servings from the monounsaturated and polyunsaturated sections of the list. Saturated fats are usually solid at room temperature, while monounsaturated and polyunsaturated fats are usually liquid at room temperature. Limit fat servings to four to six per day.

One serving has:
5 grams fat
45 calories

One serving is:
1 teaspoon margarine, butter,
    mayonnaise, or oil
1 tablespoon reduced-fat or light
    margarine or mayonnaise
1 tablespoon regular salad dressing
2 tablespoons reduced-fat or light
    salad dressing
2 tablespoons sour cream
3 tablespoons reduced-fat or light
sour cream

Fat List

Food	Quantity	Exchanges
Monounsaturated Fats		
Almond butter	1 tsp	1 fat
Avocado	2 Tbsp mashed	1 fat
Nuts		
Almonds	6 nuts	1 fat
Brazil nuts	2 medium	1 fat
Cashews	6 nuts	1 fat
Chopped nuts	1 Tbsp	1 fat
Hazelnuts (Filberts)	5 nuts	1 fat
Macadamia nuts	3 nuts	1 fat
Peanuts	10 nuts (⅓ oz)	1 fat
Pecans	4 halves	1 fat
Pine nuts, pignolia	25 nuts (1 Tbsp)	1 fat
Pistachios	15 nuts	1 fat
Soynuts	1 oz	1 fat
Nuts, mixed	5–6 nuts	1 fat
Oil (canola, olive, peanut, macadamia, grapeseed, avocado, walnut)	1 tsp	1 fat
Olives		
Green, stuffed	10 large	1 fat
Ripe, black	8 large	1 fat
Peanut butter, creamy or crunchy	1 Tbsp	1 fat
Sesame seeds	1 Tbsp	1 fat
Tahini paste (sesame paste)	2 tsp	1 fat

Food	Quantity	Exchanges
Polyunsaturated Fats		
Margarine (stick, tub, or liquid)	1 tsp	1 fat
Reduced-fat or light	1 Tbsp	1 fat
Fat-free	1 Tbsp	free
Whipped	2 tsp	1 fat
Mayonnaise	1 tsp	1 fat
Reduced-fat or light	1 Tbsp	1 fat
Miracle Whip® salad dressing	2 tsp	1 fat
Reduced-fat or light	1 Tbsp	1 fat
Oil (corn, safflower, or soybean)	1 tsp	1 fat
Salad dressings	1 Tbsp	1 fat
Reduced-fat or light	2 Tbsp	1 fat
Blue-cheese, regular	2 tsp	1 fat
Blue-cheese, reduced-fat or light	1 Tbsp	1 fat
French	1 Tbsp	1 fat
Italian	1 Tbsp	1 fat
Ranch	1 Tbsp	1 fat
Thousand Island or Russian	2 tsp	1 fat
Vinegar and oil	2 tsp	1 fat
Seeds		
Pumpkin or squash	1 Tbsp	1 fat
Soybean	1 Tbsp	1 fat
Sunflower seed kernels	1 Tbsp	1 fat
Tartar sauce	2 tsp	1 fat
Walnuts	4 halves (1 Tbsp)	1 fat

Food	Quantity	Exchanges
Saturated Fats		
Anchiote, prepared	1 tsp	1 fat
Bacon, cooked (20 slices/lb)	1 slice	1 fat
Bacon grease	1 tsp	1 fat
Butter, stick or tub	1 tsp	1 fat
Reduced-fat stick or tub	1 Tbsp	1 fat
Whipped	2 tsp	1 fat
Cheese sauce	2 Tbsp	1 fat
Cheese spread	1 Tbsp	1 fat
Chicken fat	1 tsp	1 fat
Chitterlings, boiled	2 Tbsp (½ oz)	1 fat
Coconut, shredded	2 Tbsp	1 fat
Coffee whiteners		
Nondairy liquid	2 Tbsp	1 fat
Nondairy powdered	4 tsp	1 fat
Cream, half and half	2 Tbsp	1 fat
Cream cheese	1 Tbsp (½ oz)	1 fat
Reduced-fat or light	2 Tbsp (1 oz)	1 fat
Dips		
Cream cheese-based	1 Tbsp	1 fat
Light	¼ cup	1 fat
Sour cream-based	2 Tbsp	1 fat
Gravy		
Canned	¼ cup	1 fat
Mix (as prepared)	½ cup	1 fat
Lard	1 tsp	1 fat
Liver pâté, chicken	2 Tbsp	1 fat
Neufchatel	1½ Tbsp (¾ oz)	1 fat
Shortening	1 tsp	1 fat

Food	Quantity	Exchanges
Sour cream	2 Tbsp	1 fat
Reduced-fat or light	3 Tbsp	1 fat
Whipped toppings		
Frozen	3 Tbsp	1 fat
Mix (as prepared)	5 Tbsp	1 fat

CHAPTER 8

Free Foods List

This list contains foods you can eat in addition to your meal plan without worrying about substituting or exchanging. Free foods are foods that aren't nutritionally significant – they have less than twenty calories per serving or less than five grams of carbohydrate in a serving.

One serving has:
20 calories or less per serving
5 grams or less carbohydrate per serving

Free Foods List

Food	Quantity	Exchanges
Bacon bits	1 tsp	free
Barbecue sauce	1 Tbsp	free
Bean dip	2 Tbsp	free
Bran, unprocessed	2 Tbsp	free
Brewer's yeast	2 tsp	free
Butter Buds®, dry	3 tsp	free
Candies		
Gummy bears, sugar-free	2 pieces	free
Hard candy, sugar-free	1 piece	free

Food	Quantity	Exchanges
Carbonated water, noncaloric	–	free
Catsup	1 Tbsp	free
Chewing gum, sugar-free	2 pieces	free
Bubble gum, sugar-free	1 piece	free
Chili sauce	1 Tbsp	free
Chocolate milk mix, sugar-free	1 heaping tsp	free
Club soda (not tonic or quinine water)	–	free
Cocktail sauce	1 Tbsp	free
Cocoa, dry powder, unsweetened	1 Tbsp	free
Cocoa mix, hot, no sugar added	1 Tbsp	free
Coffee	–	free
Coffee whiteners		
Nondairy liquid	1 Tbsp	free
Nondairy powdered	2 tsp	free
Light nondairy creamer	1 Tbsp	free
Coffee-Mate®, liquid	1 Tbsp	free
Cooking spray, nonstick	–	free
Cranberries, cooked without sugar	½ cup	free
Cream cheese, fat-free	1 Tbsp	free
Crystal Light® Bars (frozen)	1 bar	free
Dips, low-fat (French onion, ranch)	2 Tbsp	free
Gelatin, sugar-free, low-calorie	–	free
Gelatin, unflavored	–	free

Food	Quantity	Exchanges
Gravy		
Au jus	¼ cup	free
Canned	2 Tbsp	free
All others	2 Tbsp	free
Horseradish	3 Tbsp	free
Ice cream cones	1 cone	free
Iced tea, sugar-free	–	free
Jams and Jellies		
Dietetic	under 20 calories	free
Light	2 tsp	free
Low-sugar spreads	2 tsp	free
Spreadable fruit	1 tsp	free
Kool-Aid® or other powdered drink mix, sugar-free	–	free
Lemon juice	–	free
Lime juice	–	free
Margarine		
Reduced-fat	1 tsp	free
Fat-free	1 Tbsp	free
Mayonnaise		
Reduced-fat	1 tsp	free
Fat-free	1 Tbsp	free
Mineral water, noncaloric	–	free
Miracle Whip®		
Reduced-fat	1 tsp	free
Fat-free	1 Tbsp	free
Molly McButter® sprinkles	2 tsp	free
Mrs. Dash® herb and spice blends	1 tsp	free
Mustard	1 Tbsp	free

Food	Quantity	Exchanges
Onions	–	free
Picante sauce	2 Tbsp	free
Pickle relish	1 Tbsp	free
Pickles, dill (not sweet)		
Large	1½ large	free
Small	–	free
Pimiento	–	free
Popsicles®, sugar-free	1 pop	free
Postum® beverage	2 tsp	free
Salad dressings		
Fat-free	1 Tbsp	free
Fat-free Italian	2 Tbsp	free
Salsa, all varieties	¼ cup	free
Sauerkraut	½ cup	free
Soft drinks, diet	–	free
Soups		
Beef broth	1 cup	free
Chicken broth	½ cup	free
Consommé	¾ cup	free
Sour cream		
Fat-free	1 Tbsp	free
Reduced-fat or light	1 Tbsp	free
Soy sauce	1 Tbsp	free
Spices	–	free
Steak sauce (Heinz 57®, A1®, etc.)	1 Tbsp	free
Sugar substitutes	–	free
Syrup		
Cary's® reduced-calorie	2 Tbsp	free
Sugar-free	2 Tbsp	free

Food	Quantity	Exchanges
Tabasco sauce	1 Tbsp	free
Taco sauce	1 Tbsp	free
Tang® beverage crystals, sugar-free	–	free
Tea, sugar-free	–	free
Teriyaki sauce	1 Tbsp	free
Tomato sauce	2 Tbsp	free
Tonic water, sugar-free	–	free
Vinegar	–	free
Wine used in cooking	–	free
Whipped topping		
Cool Whip®	2 Tbsp	free
Cool Whip® Light	2 Tbsp	free
Worcestershire sauce	1 Tbsp	free
Yogurt, nonfat	2 Tbsp	free

CHAPTER 9

Combination Foods List

Many foods are combinations of foods from several of the exchange lists – pizza, lasagna, and casseroles are a few popular examples. Combination foods have the advantage of giving you nutrients from many food groups at once, but it is sometimes hard to know how to use them in your meal plan. The exchange values given are averages; the exact exchanges in a dish vary depending on the amount of each ingredient in a particular recipe.

One serving is:

Exchanges for each item:

One serving is:	Exchanges for each item:
1 cup casserole	2 starch, 2 medium fat meat, 0–1 fat
1½ cups chili	2 starch, 2 medium fat meat
2 cups Oriental entrée	2 starch, 1–2 vegetable, 1–2 medium fat meat
½ cup pasta salad or potato salad	1 starch, 1–2 fat
1 slice pizza, ⅛ large	1 starch, 1 vegetable, 1 medium fat meat, 0–1 fat
1 can (10¾ oz) chunky soup	1 starch, 1 vegetable, 2 medium fat meat

Combination Foods List

Food	Quantity	Carb Choices	Exchanges
Burrito, all varieties	1 (6 oz)	2	2 starch, 2 med. fat meat, 1 fat
Chicken à la king	1 cup	1	1 starch, 2 med. fat meat, 2 fat
Chicken and dumplings	1 cup	2	2 starch, 2 med. fat meat, 1 fat
Chicken and noodles	1 cup	2	2 starch, 2 med. fat meat, 1 fat
Chicken salad	½ cup	0	2 med. fat meat, 2 fat
Chili with beans	1 cup	2	2 starch, 2 lean meat
Chimichangas, all varieties	1 (6 oz)	2	2 starch, 1 med. fat meat, 3 fat
Chop suey	1 cup	1	1 starch, 3 med. fat meat
Chow mein (without noodles or rice)	2 cups	2	2 starch, 1 veg, 2 lean meat
Creamed chipped beef	1 cup	1	1 starch, 2 med. fat meat, 3 fat
Egg salad	½ cup	0	1 med. fat meat, 4 fat
Enchiladas	1 enchilada	2	2 starch, 1 med. fat meat, 1 fat
Entrée, less than 300 calories	1 (8 oz)	2	2 starch, 3 lean meat
Fish cake, fried	3 pieces	1	1 starch, 3 med. fat meat
French toast	2 slices	2	2 starch, 1 med. fat meat, 1 fat

Food	Quantity	Carb Choices	Exchanges
Hamburger Helper® main dishes	⅕ pkg, prepared	2	2 starch, 2 med. fat meat, 1 fat
Lasagna	1 cup	2	2 starch, 2 med. fat meat
Macaroni and cheese	1 cup	2	2 starch, 1 high fat meat
Pasta salad	½ cup	1½	1½ starch, 1–2 fat
Pizza			
Cheese or sausage	1 small slice	1	1 starch, 1 med. fat meat
Cheese, thin crust	¼ of 10" (5 oz)	2	2 starch, 2 med. fat meat, 1 fat
Meat, thin crust	¼ of 10" (5 oz)	2	2 starch, 2 med. fat meat, 2 fat
Thick crust	¼ of 10"	4	4 starch, 1 med. fat meat, 1 fat
Pot pies, all varieties	1 average (7 oz)	3	3 starch, 1 med. fat meat, 4 fat
Potato salad	½ cup	1	1 starch, 1–2 fat
Quiche, all varieties	1 slice	1½	1½ starch, 2 med. fat meat, 2 fat
Ravioli			
Beef	1 cup	2½	2½ starch, 1 med. fat meat
Cheese	1 cup	2½	2½ starch, 1 high fat meat, 1 fat
Rice-A-Roni®	1 cup	4	4 starch, 2 fat

Food	Quantity	Carb Choices	Exchanges
Salad; *see also* Chicken salad; Egg salad; Pasta salad; Potato salad; Tuna salad			
Caesar	1 serving	0	2 veg, 6 fat
Chef	1 serving	1	3 veg, 3 med. fat meat, 2 fat
Coleslaw	½ cup	0	1 veg, 2 fat
Waldorf	½ cup	0	1 fruit, 3 fat
Sandwiches			
Bacon, lettuce, tomato, mayonnaise	1 sandwich	2	2 starch, 3 fat
Chicken, lettuce, mayonnaise	1 sandwich	2	2 starch, 2 med. fat meat, 1 fat
Chicken salad	1 sandwich	2	2 starch, 2 med. fat meat, 1 fat
Club	1 sandwich	3	3 starch, 4 med. fat meat, 1 fat
Corned beef	1 sandwich	2	2 starch, 3 med. fat meat
Egg salad	1 sandwich	2	2 starch, 1 med. fat meat, 2 fat
Grilled cheese	1 sandwich	2	2 starch, 2 med. fat meat, 2 fat
Ham salad	1 sandwich	2	2 starch, 1 med. fat meat, 2 fat
Hot dog in roll	1 sandwich	1½	1½ starch, 1 high fat meat, 2 fat
Liverwurst	1 sandwich	2	2 starch, 1 high fat meat, 2 fat
Meat loaf	1 sandwich	2	2 starch, 3 med. fat meat
Peanut butter	1 sandwich	2	2 starch, 1 high fat meat, 1 fat

Food	Quantity	Carb Choices	Exchanges
Roast beef or pork with gravy	1 sandwich	2	2 starch, 2 med. fat meat, 2 fat
Submarine sandwich or hoagie	1 large	4	4 starch, 4 med. fat meat, 1 fat
Tuna salad	1 sandwich	2	2 starch, 1 med. fat meat, 2 fat
Soufflé, cheese or spinach	1½ cup	½	½ starch, 2 med. fat meat, 1 fat
Soup			
Bean soup	1 cup	1	1 starch, 1 lean meat
Broth-type soup	1 cup	1	1 starch
Chunky soup	1 can (10¾ oz)	1	1 starch, 1 veg, 1 med. fat meat
Cream soups (prepared with water)	1 cup	1	1 starch, 1 fat
Split pea (prepared with water)	½ cup	1	1 starch
Tomato (prepared with water)	1 cup	1	1 starch
Spaghetti with meatballs	1 cup	2	2 starch, 1 veg, 2 med. fat meat
Spanish rice	1 cup	3	3 starch, 1 fat
Stew, beef and vegetable	1 cup	1	1 starch, 2 med. fat meat
Tuna Helper® main dishes	⅕ pkg, prepared	2	2 starch, 2 med. fat meat
Tuna noodle casserole	1 cup	2	2 starch, 2 med. fat meat
Tuna salad	½ cup	0	2 med. fat meat, 1 fat

CHAPTER 10

Vegetarian Exchanges

Vegetarian diets can offer many health benefits. Whole grains and legumes are excellent sources of fiber, vitamins, minerals, and protein.

Many plant proteins are lacking in one or more of the essential amino acids and therefore are not complete proteins. Plant proteins can be combined with grains, milk, yogurt, cheese, or egg to provide complete proteins. Some examples of these combinations are breakfast cereal and milk, or macaroni and cheese. It's best to choose low-fat dairy foods whenever possible.

Sample Lactovegetarian Menu

Menu	Exchanges
Breakfast	
Whole wheat toast, 2 slices	2 starch
Cooked oats, ½ cup	1 starch
Orange juice, ½ cup	1 fruit
Skim milk, 1 cup	1 milk
Margarine, 2 tsp	2 fat
Snack	
Apple, 1 medium	1 fruit

Lunch

Hummus, ¼ cup	1 starch, 1 fat
Pocket bread, 1	1 starch
Yogurt, fruit-flavored, with sugar substitute, 1 cup	1 milk
Cottage cheese, ½ cup	2 lean meat
Diced tomatoes, shredded lettuce, diced onions, ½ cup	0–1 veg
Tahini, 2 tsp	1 fat

Snack

Nonfat plain yogurt, 1 cup	1 milk
Fresh fruit, ½ cup	1 fruit

Dinner

Spaghetti with lentil sauce, ½ cup pasta with 1 cup sauce	3 starch, 1 veg, 2 lean meat
Pineapple with juice, 1 slice	1 fruit
Green salad with sprouts, 1 small	1 veg
Low-calorie dressing, 2 Tbsp	1 fat

Snack

Popcorn, 3 cups	1 starch
Low-fat cheese, 1 oz	1 med. fat meat

Daily Total

Exchanges: 9 starch; 4 fruit; 3 milk; 2–3 vegetable; 4 lean meat; 1 med. fat meat; 5 fat
Calories: 1800–1900
Carbohydrate: 245 grams (54%)
Protein: 90 grams (20%)
Fat: 50 grams (26%)

Sample Vegan Menu

Menu	**Exchanges**
Breakfast	
Rye toast, 2 slices	2 starch
Scrambled tofu, ½ cup	1 med. fat meat
Fresh fruit salad, 1 cup	2 fruit
Margarine, 2 tsp	2 fat
Snack	
Apple, 1 medium	1 fruit
Lunch	
Vegetable soup, 1 bowl	2 starch
Wheat roll, 1 small	1 starch
Tossed salad, 1 small	0–1 veg
Low-fat dressing, 2 Tbsp	1 fat
Snack	
Rice cakes, 4 cakes	2 starch
Almond butter, 1 tsp	1 fat
Dinner	
Pasta, 2 cups	4 starch
Primavera with broccoli, carrots, pea pods, ½–1 cup	1–2 veg
Steamed peas, ½ cup	1 starch
French bread, 1 slice	1 starch
Margarine, 1 tsp	1 fat
Snack	
Shake of soymilk and fruit, 1½ cups	1 milk, 1 fruit, 1 fat

Daily Total
Exchanges: 13 starch; 4 fruit; 1 milk; 2–3 veg; 1 med. fat meat; 6 fat
Calories: 1800–1900
Carbohydrate: 285 grams (63%)
Protein: 60 grams (13%)
Fat: 50 grams (24%)

Vegetarian Food List

Food	Quantity	Carb Choices	Exchanges
Starch			
Amaranth, cooked	½ cup	1	1 starch
Arabic bread, Syrian bread loaf	½ of a 2-oz loaf	1	1 starch
Barley, cooked	⅓ cup	1	1 starch
Brewer's yeast	3 Tbsp	1	1 starch, 1 lean meat
Buckwheat flour, dark or light	3 Tbsp	1	1 starch
Buckwheat groats (kasha), cooked	½ cup	1	1 starch
Bulgur, cooked	½ cup (2 Tbsp dry)	1	1 starch
Carob flour	2 Tbsp	1	1 starch
Couscous, cooked	⅓ cup	1	1 starch

Food	Quantity	Carb Choices	Exchanges
Falafel, 2" across	3 patties	1	1 starch, 1 med. fat meat, 2 fat
Hummus	¼ cup	1	1 starch, 1 fat
Millet, cooked	¼ cup	1	1 starch
Miso	3 Tbsp	1	1 starch
	½ cup	2½	2½ starch, 1 med. fat meat
Oatmeal, cooked	½ cup	1	1 starch
Pasta	½ cup	1	1 starch
Pasta and tomato sauce	2 cups	4	4 starch, 2 veg, 1 fat
Pocket/Pita bread			
4½" across	1 pocket/pita	1	1 starch
6½" across	½ pocket/pita (1 oz)	1	1 starch
Rice			
Brown, cooked	⅓ cup	1	1 starch
White, cooked	⅓ cup	1	1 starch
Wild, cooked	½ cup	1	1 starch
Rice cakes, all flavors			
4" across	2 cakes	1	1 starch
Mini	½ oz	1	1 starch
Rye flour	3 Tbsp	1	1 starch
Soybean flour	½ cup	1	1 starch, 2 med. fat meat
Low-fat	½ cup	1	1 starch, 3 lean meat
Tabouli	¼ cup	1½	1½ starch, 1 fat
Tempeh	½ cup	1	1 starch, 2 med. fat meat
Wheat berries, cooked	⅔ cup	1	1 starch

Food	Quantity	Carb Choices	Exchanges
Wheat bran, toasted	⅓ cup	1	1 starch
Wheat germ, toasted	¼ cup	1	1 starch, 1 very lean meat
Vegetables with braised tofu	2 cups	1	1 starch, 1 veg, 1 med. fat meat, 2 fat
Vegetarian egg rolls with sweet and sour sauce	3 mini	1½	1½ starch, 1 veg
Milk			
Goat milk	1 cup	1	1 milk, 1½ fat
Kefir	1 cup	1	1 milk, 1½ fat
Soy milk; *see also* Meat Substitutes below			
Light	1 cup	1	1 milk
Regular	1 cup	1½	1½ milk, 1 fat
Yogurt, fruit-flavored, sweetened with a sugar substitute	8 oz	1	1 milk
Yogurt, nonfat plain	6 oz	1	1 milk
Vegetable; *see also* Vegetable List			
Bamboo shoots, cooked	½ cup	0	1 veg
Carrot juice	¼ cup	0	1 veg
Seaweed, cooked	½ cup	0	1 veg
Sprouts (alfalfa, bean, mung, soy)	1 cup raw or ¾ cup cooked	0	1 veg
Water chestnuts, canned	6 whole	0	1 veg
Meat Substitutes			
Beans, dried, cooked			
Black beans (turtle beans)	1 cup	2	2 starch, 1 very lean meat

Food	Quantity	Carb Choices	Exchanges
Broad beans (fava beans)	⅔ cup	2	2 starch, 1 very lean meat
Calico beans	1 cup	2	2 starch, 1 very lean meat
Garbanzo beans (chickpeas)	⅔ cup	2	2 starch, 1 very lean meat
Kidney beans	1 cup	2	2 starch, 1 very lean meat
Lima beans	1 cup	2	2 starch, 1 very lean meat
Mung beans	1 cup	2	2 starch, 1 very lean meat
Navy beans	⅔ cup	2	2 starch, 1 very lean meat
Pinto beans	⅔ cup	2	2 starch, 1 very lean meat

Cheese; *see* Meat and Meat Substitutes List

La Loma* products

Food	Quantity	Carb Choices	Exchanges
Big franks, canned	1 frank	0	2 lean meat
Chicken, fried, frozen	1 piece (2 oz)	0	2 med. fat meat, 1 fat
Corn dogs, frozen	1 corn dog	1	1 starch, 2 med. fat meat
Griddle steak, frozen	1 steak (2 oz)	0	2 lean meat
Nuteena, canned	1 slice (½" thick)	0	1 med. fat meat, 2 fat
Savory meatballs, frozen	7 meatballs	0	1 veg, 3 lean meat
Swiss steak, canned	1 piece	0	1 veg, 2 med. fat meat
Vege-burger, canned	½ cup	0	3 lean meat

Food	Quantity	Carb Choices	Exchanges
Lentils	1 cup	2	2 starch, 1 lean meat
Morningstar Farms® products			
Breakfast links, frozen	2 links	0	1 med. fat meat
Breakfast patty, frozen	1 patty	0	1 high fat meat
Scramblers, frozen	¼ cup	0	1 lean meat
Natto	½ cup	1	1 starch, 2 med. fat meat
Natural Touch® products			
Lentil rice loaf, frozen	2½" slice	0	1 med. fat meat, 1 fat
Vegetarian chili, canned	⅔ cup	1	1 starch, 2 med. fat meat
Nuts			
Almonds	¼ cup (1 oz)	0	1 medium fat meat, 2 fat
Brazil nuts	¼ cup (1 oz)	0	1 high fat meat, 2 fat
Butternuts	¼ cup (1 oz)	0	1 medium fat meat, 2 fat
Peanut butter	1 Tbsp	0	1 high fat meat
Peanuts, roasted	¼ cup (1 oz)	0	1 medium fat meat, 2 fat
Pecans	¼ cup (1 oz)	0	1 medium fat meat, 2 fat
Pignolias, pine nuts	2 Tbsp	0	1 medium fat meat, 2 fat
Pistachio	47 nuts (1 oz)	0	1 medium fat meat, 2 fat
Walnuts	16–20 halves (1 oz)	0	1 medium fat meat, 2 fat

Food	Quantity	Carb Choices	Exchanges
Peas, dried, cooked			
Black-eyed peas	1 cup	2	2 starch, 1 lean meat
Split peas	⅔ cup	2	2 starch, 1 lean meat
Seeds			
Pumpkin or squash	¼ cup	0	1 medium fat meat, 2 fat
Sesame	¼ cup	0	1 medium fat meat, 2 fat
Sunflower	¼ cup	0	1 medium fat meat, 2 fat
Sunflowers with hulls	½ cup	0	1 medium fat meat, 2 fat
Soybeans, cooked	½ cup	½	½ starch, 1 med. fat meat
Soybean flour	½ cup	1	1 starch, 2 med. fat meat
Low-fat	½ cup	1	1 starch, 3 lean meat
Soy grits, raw	2 Tbsp	0	1 lean meat
Soy milk, fortified	1 cup	1½	½ other carb, 1 med. fat meat
Tempeh	¼ cup	0	1 med. fat meat
	½ cup	1	1 starch, 2 med. fat meat
Tofu	½ cup	0	1 med. fat meat
Tofu hot dog	1 hot dog	0	1 med. fat meat
Vegetable protein, textured	¾ oz	½	½ starch, 1 lean meat
Worthington Foods® products			
Bolono, frozen	2 slices	0	1 lean meat

Food	Quantity	Carb Choices	Exchanges
Chicken, frozen	2 slices	0	1 med. fat meat, 1 fat
Chili, canned	⅔ cup	1	1 starch, 1 med. fat meat, 1 fat
Choplets, canned	2 slices	0	2 lean meat
Corned beef, frozen	4 slices	½	½ starch, 1 med. fat meat
Country stew	9½ oz can	1	1 starch, 1 veg, 1 med. fat meat, 1 fat
Cutlets, canned	1½ slices	0	2 lean meat
Dinner roast, frozen	2 slices (3 oz)	0	1 high fat meat
Non-meat balls, canned	3 pieces	0	1 high fat meat
Prime stakes	1 piece	½	½ starch, 1 med. fat meat, 1 fat
Prosage links, frozen	2 links	0	1 high fat meat
Salami, meatless, frozen	2 slices	½	½ starch, 1 lean meat
Smoked beef, frozen	3 slices	½	½ starch, 1 med. fat meat
Smoked turkey, frozen	4 slices	0	2 lean meat
Tuno, frozen	2 oz	0	1 high fat meat
Turkee slices, canned	2 slices	0	1 med. fat meat, 1 fat
Vegetable skallops, canned	½ cup	0	2 lean meat
Vegetarian beef or chicken pie, frozen	1 pie	3	3 starch, 4 fat
Vegetarian burger, canned	½ cup	½	½ starch, 2 lean meat
Vegetarian egg roll	1 large	1	1 starch, 1 veg, 1 fat

Food	Quantity	Carb Choices	Exchanges
Wham, frozen	3 slices	0	2 med. fat meat
Fat			
Almond paste	2 tsp	0	1 fat
Bacon, simulated meat product	2 strips	0	1 fat
Lecithin	2 tsp	0	1 fat
Tahini paste	2 tsp	0	1 fat
Tofu cream cheese	1 Tbsp	0	1 fat
Free			
Carob powder	1 Tbsp	0	free
Sprouts	½ cup	0	free

CHAPTER 11

Asian Food Exchanges

Asian cuisines offer many selections that fit easily into a healthy diet. Cooking methods tend to be low fat, such as steaming, boiling, or stir-frying in a small amount of hot oil. Milk and cheese are rarely used, and only small portions of meat or seafood are used. However, certain items signal caution.

Japanese

Good Choices

Nabemono (boiled)
    or yakimono
    (broiled) dishes
Combinations of grilled
    meats or seafood
    and vegetables
Kayaku goban
Miso and bean soups
Sashimi or sushi
Shabu shabu
Shumai
Soba or udon noodles
Steamed rice

Go Easy

Agemono
Chicken katsu
Fried tofu
Sukiyaki
Tempura
Tonkatsu
Yakitori
Yosenabe

Chinese

Good Choices
Hot and sour shrimp
Wonton soup
Steamed dumplings
Chicken chow mein
Chicken and beef
    chop suey
Chicken or vegetable
    lo mein
Chicken or beef teriyaki
Moo shu shrimp
    or chicken
Stir-fried meat with
    vegetables
Steamed rice
Lobster, hoisin, black bean,
    and plum sauces
Fortune cookies

Go Easy
Fried noodles
Egg foo yong
Crispy or batter-coated foods
Egg rolls
Fried wontons
Sweet and sour chicken
Cashew chicken
Barbecued spare ribs
Beef or pork fried rice

Thai

Good Choices
Hang mung poo
Hot and sour soup
Po tak
Stir-fried noodles
    and sprouts
Sautéed ginger beef
    or chicken

Go Easy
Curries and soups based on
    coconut milk
Crispy or deep-fried Thai
    rolls or tofu
Crispy fried rice
Coconut ice cream or
    puddings
Peanut sauces

Sample Japanese Meal

Menu

	Exchanges
Su-udon soup, 1 cup	1 starch, 1 fat
Donburi, oyako, 1½ cup	3 starch, 1 veg, 1 med. fat meat
Teriyaki salmon, 4 oz	4 lean meat
Steamed rice, ⅓ cup	1 starch

Meal Total

Exchanges: 5 starch; 1 veg; 4 lean meat; 1 med. fat meat; 1 fat

Calories: 750

Carbohydrate: 80 grams (43%)

Protein: 45 grams (24%)

Fat: 28 grams (33%)

Sample Chinese Meal

Menu

	Exchanges
Wonton soup, 1 cup	1 starch, 1 fat
Yu hsiang chicken, 1½ cups	1 veg, 2 med. fat meat
Beef with broccoli and black mushroom,	1 veg, 2 med. fat meat
Steamed white rice, ⅔ cup	2 starch
Fortune cookie, 1 cookie	1 starch or 1 other carb

Meal Total

Exchanges: 4 starch (or 3 starch and 1 other carb); 2 veg; 4 med. fat meat; 1 fat

Calories: 700

Carbohydrate: 70 grams (40%)

Protein: 45 grams (25%)

Fat: 30 grams (35%)

Sample Thai Meal

Menu	Exchanges
Tom yum koong, 1 cup	1 starch
Tai chicken, 1 cup	1 veg, 2 lean meat, 1 fat
Poy sian, 1 cup	1 veg, 2 lean meat, 1 fat
Steamed rice, 1 cup	3 starch
Hot tea	free

Meal Total

Exchanges: 4 starch; 2 veg; 4 lean meat; 2 fat
Calories: 700
Carbohydrate: 70 grams (41%)
Protein: 45 grams (26%)
Fat: 25 grams (33%)

Asian Food List

Food	Quantity	Carb Choices	Exchanges
Starch			
Adzuki beans, cooked	⅓ cup	1	1 starch
Almond cookie	2 medium	1	1 starch or 1 other carb
Arrowroot starch	2 Tbsp	1	1 starch
Bow (Chinese steamed dough)	1 small	1	1 starch
Cellophane noodles, cooked	¾ cup	1	1 starch
Chinese noodles	⅓ cup	1	1 starch
Chow mein noodles	½ cup	1	1 starch, 1 fat
Chestnuts	4 large	1	1 starch
Congee rice soup	¾ cup	1	1 starch
Cornstarch	2 Tbsp	1	1 starch
Egg roll wrapper	2 wrappers	1	1 starch
Fortune cookie	2 cookies	1	1 starch or 1 other carb
Fried rice	⅓ cup	1	1 starch, 1 fat
	1 cup	3	3 starch, 3 fat
Ginkgo seeds	½ cup	1	1 starch
Glutinous rice (Sticky rice)	⅓ cup	1	1 starch
Lotus root	10 slices	1	1 starch
Miso	3 Tbsp	1	1 starch
	½ cup	2½	2½ starch, 1 med. fat meat
Mung beans, cooked	⅓ cup	1	1 starch
Mung bean noodles	¾ cup	1	1 starch
Poi (taro), cooked	⅓ cup	1	1 starch
Red beans, cooked	⅓ cup	1	1 starch

Food	Quantity	Carb Choices	Exchanges
Rice, cooked, loosely packed	⅓ cup	1	1 starch
Rice noodles, vermicelli, cooked	½ cup	1	1 starch
Rice soup	¾ cup	1	1 starch
Soba noodles	½ cup	1	1 starch
Su-udon soup	1 cup	1	1 starch, 1 fat
Tom yum koong soup	1 cup	1	1 starch
Udon noodles	½ cup	1	1 starch
Wonton wrappers, 3" x 3"	4 wrappers	1	1 starch
Wonton, fried	3 medium	1	1 starch, 3 fat
Wheat fritters	1 medium	1	1 starch
Yard-long beans, pods, and seeds	1 cup	1	1 starch
Fruit			
Apple pear (Asian pear)	1 medium	1	1 fruit
Carambola	1½ medium	1	1 fruit
Dried salted apricots	6 halves	1	1 fruit
Guava	1 medium	1	1 fruit
Kumquats	5 medium	1	1 fruit
Longans	30 medium	1	1 fruit
Canned	¾ cup	1	1 fruit
Loquats	12 fruits	1	1 fruit
Lychees, fresh or dried	10 medium	1	1 fruit
Canned	½ cup	1	1 fruit
Mango	½ medium	1	1 fruit
Papaya	½ fruit	1	1 fruit
Persimmon, Japanese	½ medium	1	1 fruit
Pomelo	¾ cup	1	1 fruit
Red dates	6 medium	1	1 fruit

Food	Quantity	Carb Choices	Exchanges
Milk			
Coconut milk	1 cup	½	½ milk, 7 fat
Light	1 cup	½	½ milk, 3 fat
Soy milk	1 cup	1½	1½ milk, 1 fat
Vegetable			
Arrowroot	1 (2" across)	0	1 veg
Bamboo shoots, canned	½ cup	0	1 veg
Bean sprouts	1 cup raw or ¾ cup cooked	0	1 veg
Bitter melon	½ cup	0	1 veg
Bok choy, cooked	1 cup	0	1 veg
Button or straw mushrooms	½ cup	0	1 veg
Chayote	½ cup	0	1 veg
Chinese cabbage	2 cups raw or 1 cup cooked	0	1 veg
Chinese spinach, cooked	½ cup	0	1 veg
Corn, baby, canned	½ cup	0	1 veg
Daikon (Chinese radish)	1 cup	0	1 veg
Fuzzy melon	½ cup	0	1 veg
Ginger root	¼ cup	0	1 veg
Kohlrabi	⅔ cup	0	1 veg
Leeks (Chinese onion)	½ cup or 2 medium	0	1 veg
Miso	1 Tbsp	0	1 veg
Mushrooms, dried, black	¼ cup	0	1 veg
Mustard leaves	½ cup	0	1 veg
Nori	1 small sheet	0	1 veg
Peas or peapods	½ cup	0	1 veg
Seaweed laver, soaked	½ cup	0	1 veg

Food	Quantity	Carb Choices	Exchanges
Seahair, soaked	½ cup	0	1 veg
Taro root	¼ cup	0	1 veg
Meat/Meat Substitutes			
Albalone	1 oz	0	1 lean meat
Chicken wings	1 wing	0	1 lean meat
Chinese sausage	½ sausage (1 oz)	0	1 high fat meat
Duck egg, preserved	1 egg	0	1 high fat meat
Duck feet	3 medium	0	1 med. fat meat
Eel	1 oz	0	1 high fat meat
Fish maw	2 oz	0	1 med. fat meat
Horse beans (broad beans)	⅔ cup	2	2 starch, 1 lean meat
Octopus	2 oz	0	1 lean meat
Oxtail	1 oz	0	1 med. fat meat
Pork feet	2 oz	0	1 high fat meat
Poy sian	1 cup	0	1 veg, 2 lean meat, 1 fat
Red mung beans	⅔ cup	2	2 starch, 1 lean meat
Scallops, dried	1 large	0	1 lean meat
Shrimp, dried	10 shrimp (½ oz)	0	1 lean meat
Squid	1 oz	0	1 very lean meat
Tofu	½ cup (4 oz)	0	1 med. fat meat

Food	Quantity	Carb Choices	Exchanges
Fat			
Chicken fat or pork fat	1 tsp	0	1 fat
Coconut, grated	2 Tbsp	0	1 fat
Coconut milk	2 Tbsp	0	1 fat
Light	¼ cup	0	1 fat
Macadamia nuts	3 medium	0	1 fat
Pork, cured	1" cube	0	1 fat
Sesame or peanut oil	1 tsp	0	1 fat
Sesame paste	2 tsp	0	1 fat
Sesame seeds	1 Tbsp	0	1 fat
Watermelon seeds	⅓ oz	0	1 fat
Free Foods			
Coriander	–	0	free
Curry	–	0	free
Dipping sauce	2 Tbsp	0	free
Fish sauce	–	0	free
Fortune cookie	1 cookie	0	free
	2 cookies	1	1 other carb
Garlic	–	0	free
Ginger	–	0	free
Green onion	–	0	free
Hot mustard	–	0	free
Miso dressing	2 Tbsp	0	free
Soy sauce (tamari)	–	0	free
Star anise	–	0	free
Sweet and sour sauce	1 Tbsp	0	free

Food	Quantity	Carb Choices	Exchanges
Combination Dishes			
Beef and vegetables	2 cups	2	2 starch, 1 veg, 2 med. fat meat
Cashew nut chicken	1 cup	1	1 starch, 2 med. fat meat, 4 fat
Chicken and vegetables	2 cups	2	2 starch, 1 veg, 2 lean meat
Chinese broccoli with beef or pork	1 cup	1	1 starch, 3 fat meat, 2–3 fat
Chop suey	2 cups	2	2 starch, 3–4 med. fat meat, 1–2 fat
Chow luny aas	¾ cup	0	3 med. fat meat, 1 fat
Chow mein (beef, pork, or chicken)	2 cups	2	2 starch, 1 veg, 2–3 med. fat meat, 1–2 fat
Crispy shrimp	1 cup	2	2 starch, 3 med. fat meat, 4–5 fat
Dim sum			
Gow-Gee	3 pieces	1	1 starch, 1 med. fat meat
Har-Gow	3 pieces	½	½ starch, ½ med. fat meat
Siu-Mai	2 pieces	½	½ starch, 1 med. fat meat
War-Tip	2 pieces	½	½ starch, 1 med. fat meat
Donburi, oyako	1½ cups	3	3 starch, 1 veg, 1 med. fat meat
Egg drop soup	1 cup	0	½ med. fat meat
Egg flower soup	2 cups	0	1 med. fat meat

Food	Quantity	Carb Choices	Exchanges
Egg foo yong	1 medium patty	0	1 veg, 2 med. fat meat, 2 fat
Egg foo yong sauce	¼ cup	0	1 veg
Egg roll (chicken, pork, or shrimp)	1 small	1	1 starch, 1 med. fat meat, 2 fat
Fried rice (rice, meat, eggs, and onion)	1 cup	2	2 starch, 1 med. fat meat, 2 fat
Fung gawn aar	1 cup	0	3 med. fat meat, 2 fat
Hot and sour soup	1 cup	0	1 veg, 1 med. fat meat
Mock duck	1 cup	1	1 starch, 2 lean meat
Moo goo gai pan	2 cups	1	1 starch, 1 veg, 2–3 med. fat meat, 0–1 fat
Moo shi shrimp	2 pancakes with 1 cup filling	1	1 starch, 2 veg, 2 med. fat meat, 1 fat
Mum yee mein	1 cup	2	2 starch, 2 med. fat meat, 1 fat
Peking ravioli, steamed	2 medium	1	1 starch, 1 med. fat meat, 1 fat
Pepper steak	1 cup	1	1 starch, 3 med. fat meat, 1 veg
Ramaki	2 pieces	0	1 med. fat meat, 1 fat
Rice soup	¾ cup	1	1 starch
Shiu mi	2 pieces	½	½ starch, ½ fat
Shrimp and vegetables	2 cups	2	2 starch, 1 veg, 2 lean meat

Food	Quantity	Carb Choices	Exchanges
Shrimp with broccoli and mushrooms	1 cup	0	1 veg, 2 med. fat meat, 1 fat
Siumoni soup	1 cup	0	1 veg
Snow pea shrimp or chicken	1 cup	1	1 starch, 2–3 med. fat meat, 2 fat
Sukiyaki	1½ cup	0	3 med. fat meat, 1 fat
Sweet and sour pork or shrimp	1 cup	4	4 starch, 2 med. fat meat, 1–2 fat
Tai chicken	1 cup	0	1 veg, 2 lean meat, 1 fat
Vegetable lo mein noodles	1½ cup	3	3 starch, 1 veg, 1 fat
Wonton, boiled	4 wonton	1	1 starch, 1 med. fat meat, 1 fat
Wonton soup	2 wonton and 1 cup broth	1	1 starch, 1 fat
Yaki-udon soup	1 cup	0	1 veg, 1 fat
Yu hsiang chicken with ⅓ cup rice	1 cup	1	1 starch, 1 veg, 2 med. fat meat

CHAPTER 12

Exchanges Mexican Style

From simple snacks like chips and salsa to upscale restaurant meals, foods from Mexico and the American Southwest have a central place in our culinary melting pot. Using grains, beans, and chiles as staples, south-of-the-border dishes can add spice to your meals along with good nutrition. To fire up your food plan, try some of the dishes influenced by our neighbors to the south!

Good Choices

Arroz con pollo (remove the skin)
Bean, vegetable, chicken, or fish soft burritos
Beans or refried beans (without lard)
Black bean soup
Ceviche
Chicken enchiladas
Chicken, beef, or shrimp fajitas
Chicken, seafood, or bean enchiladas
Gazpacho soup

Go Easy

Carne asada
Cheese
Chili con queso
Chile rellenos
Chimichangas
Chorizo
Fried dishes
Fried ice cream
Fried tamales
Guacamole
Huevos reales
Mole polo
Nachos
Refried beans (with lard)

Good Choices	*Go Easy*
Hot sauce or chili sauce	Sopapillas
Mexican rice	Sour cream
Plain yogurt and yogurt sauces	
Red beans and rice	
Salsa, salsa verde, or picante sauce	
Shrimp or fish Veracruz	
Soft chicken tacos	
Tomato, onion, and avocado salad (with a squeeze of lemon juice)	

Sample Mexican Meal

Menu	**Exchanges**
Black bean soup, 1 cup	2 starch
Chicken enchilada, 1 enchilada	2 starch, 2 med. fat meat, 1–2 fat
Beef taco, 1 taco	1 starch, 1 med. fat meat, 1 fat
Spanish rice, ½ cup	1 starch, 1 veg

Meal Total

Exchanges: 6 starch; 1 veg; 3 med. fat meat; 2–3 fat
Calories: 800
Carbohydrate: 95 grams (46%)
Protein: 40 grams (20%)
Fat: 31 grams (34%)

Mexican Food List

Food	Quantity	Carb Choices	Exchanges
Starch			
Amaranth, cooked	½ cup	1	1 starch
Beans			
Black, boiled or canned	½ cup	1	1 starch
Pinto or kidney, boiled or canned	⅓ cup	1	1 starch
	1 cup	2	2 starch, 1 very lean meat
Refried	⅓ cup	1	1 starch, 1 fat
Black bean soup	1 cup	2	2 starch
Bolillo	1½" piece	1	1 starch
Breadfruit	2 wedges (2"x1")	1	1 starch
Cassava	½ cup	1	1 starch
Corn chips	1 cup (1 oz)	1	1 starch, 2 fat
Cornbread	2" square	1	1 starch, 1 fat
Hard roll			
3" across	1 roll	1	1 starch
6" across	⅓ roll	1	1 starch
Hominy	½ cup	1	1 starch
"Hops" bread	1 small	1	1 starch
Jicama	1 cup	1	1 starch
Malanga	⅓ cup	1	1 starch
Masa harina	2 Tbsp	1	1 starch
Plantain, mature, cooked	⅓ medium	1	1 starch
Spanish rice	½ cup	1	1 starch, 1 fat
Taco shell, 6" across	2 shells	1	1 starch, 1 fat

Food	Quantity	Carb Choices	Exchanges
Tortillas			
Corn, 6" across	1 tortilla	1	1 starch
Flour, 7–8" across	1 tortilla	1	1 starch
Flour, 12" across	1 tortilla	2	2 starch
Tortilla chips, fried	6–12 chips (1 oz)	1	1 starch, 2 fat
Vermicelli	½ cup	1	1 starch
Yam, white	½ cup	1	1 starch
Yautia (tannier)	1 small	1	1 starch
Boiled	½ cup	1	1 starch
Fruit			
Apple banana	½ medium	1	1 fruit
Cactus fruit	1 medium	1	1 fruit
Cherimoya	½ small	1	1 fruit
Coco plum	1 medium	1	1 fruit
Guava	1 medium	1	1 fruit
Guava nectar	½ cup	1	1 fruit
Mamey	½ medium	1	1 fruit
Mango	½ small	1	1 fruit
Papaya	1 cup cubes	1	1 fruit
Sapota (Custard apple)	1 small	1	1 fruit
Other Carbohydrates			
Flan (Mexican custard)	1 cup	3	3 other carb, 3 fat
Pan dulce (sweet bread)	1 (4½" across)	4	4 other carb, 1 fat
Sopa (sweet Spanish bread soup)	1 cup	4	4 other carb, 2 fat

Food	Quantity	Carb Choices	Exchanges
Vegetable			
Amaranth, cooked	½ cup	0	1 veg
Calabazita, cooked	½ cup	0	1 veg
Chayote	½ cup	0	1 veg
Cactus leaves (Nopales)	½ cup	0	1 veg
Gazpacho	½ cup	0	1 veg
Jalapeno peppers	4 peppers	0	1 veg
Jicama	½ cup	0	1 veg
Okra	½ cup	0	1 veg
Spanish sauce	½ cup	1	1 veg
Tomatoes, green	½ cup or 2 small	0	1 veg
Verdolages (purslane)	½ cup	0	1 veg
Meat			
Chorizo, beef or pork	1 oz	0	1 high fat meat, 1 fat
Goat meat	4 small cubes	0	1 med. fat meat
Queso (cheese) Jalisco, Fresco, or Mexican	1 oz	0	1 med. fat meat
Skirt steak	1 oz	0	1 lean meat
Fat			
Ackee	3 pieces	0	1 fat
Avocado	⅛ medium	0	1 fat
Ghee	1 tsp	0	1 fat
Guacamole	2 Tbsp	0	1 fat
Sofrito	2 tsp	0	1 fat
Free Foods			
Chile peppers	–	0	free
Cilantro, fresh	–	0	free

Food	Quantity	Carb Choices	Exchanges
Salsa	¼ cup	0	free
Taco sauce	–	0	free
Combination Foods			
Arroz con pollo	¾ cup	1	1 starch, 2 med. fat meat, 1 fat
Beef cubes in brown gravy	1 cup	1	1 starch, 2 med. fat meat, 1 fat
Burrito de carne			
7" across	1 burrito	2	2 starch, 2 med. fat meat, 1 fat (If deep-fried, add extra fat)
9" across	1 burrito	3	3 starch, 3 med. fat meat, 1 fat
Burrito de frijoles refritos			
7" across	1 burrito	3	3 starch, 1 med. fat meat, 2 fat (If deep-fried, add 1–2 extra fat)
9" across	1 burrito	4	4 starch, 1½ med. fat meat, 2 fat
Chicken and yellow squash	¾ cup	0	2 lean meat, 1 veg, 2 fat
Chili con carne			
With beans	1 cup	2	2 starch, 2 med. fat meat
Without beans	1 cup	½	½ starch, 3 med. fat meat
Chili rellenos	1 pepper (7" long)	2	2 starch, 1 veg, 2 med. fat meat, 3 fat

Food	Quantity	Carb Choices	Exchanges
Chili verde	1 cup	1	1 starch, 1 veg, 3 med. fat meat, 2 fat
Chimichangas, all varieties	1 (6 oz)	3	3 starch, 2 med. fat meat, 2 fat
Corn fritters	1 (3" across)	1	1 starch, 2 med. fat meat, 1 fat
Enchiladas, beef or chicken	1 enchilada	2	2 starch, 2 med. fat meat, 1–2 fat
Enchiladas, cheese	1 enchilada	2	2 starch, 1–2 med. fat meat, 3–4 fat
Enchirito	1 medium	2	2 starch, 2 med. fat meat, 1 fat
Ensalada de aquacite	½ cup	0	1 veg, 3 fat
Fajitas	2 fajitas	4	4 starch, 3 med. fat meat, 2 fat
Flauta	1 flauta	1	1 starch, 1 med. fat meat
Frijoles with cheese	1 cup	2	2 starch, 1 med. fat meat, 2 fat
Menudo	½ cup	0	1 lean meat
Mexican rice	½ cup	1	1 starch, 1 veg, 1 fat
Mexican squash with beef	½ cup	0	1 med. fat meat, 1 veg, 1 fat
Nachos (cheese)	6–8 nachos	2½	2½ starch, 1 high fat meat, 2 fat
Nachos (cheese, beans, beef)	6–8 nachos	3½	3½ starch, 2 med. fat meat, 3 fat

Food	Quantity	Carb Choices	Exchanges
Picadillo	¾ cup	1	1 starch, 2 med. fat meat, 2 fat
Quesadillas	1 quesadilla	2	2 starch, 2 med. fat meat, 1 fat
Spanish rice	½ cup	1	1 starch, 1 veg
Taco			
Small (6–7")	1 taco	1	1 starch, 1–2 med. fat meat, 1 fat
Large	1 taco	3	3 starch, 3 med. fat meat, 3 fat
Taco, open	1 taco	1	1 starch, 3 med. fat meat, 1 veg
Taco salad	1 large	3	4 starch, 1 veg, 3 med. fat meat, 5 fat
Tamales, beef (with sauce)	2 small or 1 large	2	2 starch, 1–2 med. fat meat, 2 fat
Tostada			
Bean	1 small	2	2 starch, 2 fat
Beef	1 small	1	1 starch, 1 med. fat meat, 1 fat
Beef and cheese	1 large	1½	1½ starch, 2 med. fat meat, 1 fat
Beef, cheese, and beans	1 large	2	2 starch, 2 med. fat meat, 2 fat
Beef, cheese, and beans with guacamole	1 large	2	2 starch, 2 med. fat meat, 3 fat
Vermicelli or rice with beef	1 cup	2	2 starch, 2 med. fat meat, 1 fat

CHAPTER 13

Exchanges Italiano

For some of our favorite foods, such as pizza and spaghetti, Americans are beholden to Italy. One of the most enjoyable aspects of Italian cooking is its diversity, which reflects the country's varied geography and climate. From Genoa in the north to Sicily in the south, Italy's regions use their native ingredients to create a dizzying and delicious array of dishes.

Good Choices
Bruschetta
Chicken cacciatore
Chicken marsala
Italian ice
Linguine with white or
    red clam sauce
Minestrone Soup
Mussels marinara
Pasta primavera
Veal cacciatore
Zita bolognese
Zuppa de pesce

Go Easy
Alfredo sauce
Cannelloni
Cannoli
Carbonara sauce
Cream sauces
Eggplant or chicken
    parmigiana
Fettuccine alfredo
Fried calamari
Lasagna
Prosciutto
Salami
Shrimp scampi

Sample Italian Meal

Menu	Exchanges
Minestrone, 1 cup	1 starch, 1 fat
Italian bread with garlic butter, 1 slice	1 starch, 1 fat
Veal cacciatore, 1 cutlet with sauce	3 starch, 3 lean meat, 1 fat
House salad with Italian dressing, 1 side salad	1 veg, 0–1 fat
Italian ice, ½ cup	1½ other carb

Meal Total

Exchanges: 5 starch; 1 veg; 1½ other carb; 3 lean meat; 3–4 fat
Calories: 850
Carbohydrate: 100 grams (46%)
Protein: 40 grams (21%)
Fat: 30 grams (33%)

Italian Food List

Food	Quantity	Carb Choices	Exchanges
Starch			
Alfredo sauce	½ cup	1½	1½ starch, 1 med. fat meat, 2 fat
Bolognese sauce	½ cup	1	1 starch, 1 fat
Gnocchi	2 small	1	1 starch
Italian bread	1 slice (1 oz)	1	1 starch
Italian bread with garlic butter	1 slice (1 oz)	1	1 starch, 1–2 fat
Marinara sauce	½ cup	1	1 starch, 1 fat
With mushrooms	½ cup	1	1 starch, 1 fat
With meat	½ cup	1	1 starch, 1 fat
Meat-flavored or mushroom spaghetti sauce	½ cup	1	1 starch, 1 fat
Minestrone soup	1 cup	1	1 starch, 1 fat
Pasta	½ cup	1	1 starch
Red clam sauce	1 cup	1	1 starch, 1 fat
Spaghetti sauce	½ cup	1	1 starch
Spaghetti sauce with meat	½ cup	1	1 starch, 1 med. fat meat
Vermicelli soup	1 cup	1	1 starch
Other Carbohydrates			
Italian ice	½ cup	1½	1½ other carb
Spumoni	½ cup	1	1 other carb, 2 fat

Food	Quantity	Carb Choices	Exchanges
Vegetable			
Italian green beans	½ cup	0	1 veg
Pizza sauce	¼ cup	0	1 veg
Ratatouille	½ cup	0	1 veg, 1 fat
Tomato paste	2 Tbsp	0	1 veg
Tomato puree	¼ cup	0	1 veg
Tomato sauce	⅓ cup	0	1 veg
Meat			
Italian sausage	1 oz	0	1 high fat meat
Meatballs	1 meatball (2" across)	0	1 med. fat meat
Prosciutto (Italian ham)	1 oz	0	1 med. fat meat
Veal cutlet	1 oz	0	1 lean meat
White clam sauce	½ cup	0	1 high fat meat
Fat			
Italian dressing	1 Tbsp	0	1 fat
Olive oil	1 Tbsp	0	2 fat
Pesto sauce	2 Tbsp (1 oz)	0	3 fat
Combination Dishes			
Antipasto	1 serving	0	2 veg, 2 high fat meat, 1 fat
Cannelloni	4 medium	2	2 starch, 3 med. fat meat, 2–3 fat
Cannelloni Florentine	4 medium	2	2 starch, 2 med. fat meat, 2 fat
Chicken cacciatore	½ small breast	1	1 starch, 3 lean meat, 1 fat

Food	Quantity	Carb Choices	Exchanges
Chicken parmigiana with noodles	½ small breast +1 cup noodles	1	1 starch, 1 veg, 3 lean meat, 1 fat
Chicken or turkey tetrazzini	1 cup	2	2 starch, 1 veg, 2 med. fat meat
Eggplant parmigiana	1 cup	1	1 starch, 1 veg, 2 med. fat meat, 1 fat
Fettuccine alfredo	1½ cup	2	2 starch, 6 fat
Fettuccine primavera	1½ cup	2	2 starch, 1 veg, 1 med. fat meat, 2 fat
Fettuccine with chicken	1 cup	2	2 starch, 2 med. fat meat, 1 fat
Lasagna			
Cheese or beef	3 x 4" piece	1	1 starch, 1 veg, 2 med. fat meat
Sausage	3 x 4" piece	2	2 starch, 3 med. fat meat, 3 fat
Linguini with white clam sauce	1 cup	3	3 starch, 1 med. fat meat, 2–3 fat
Manicotti			
With ricotta and tomato sauce	2 shells	3	3 starch, 2 med. fat meat, 2 fat
With ricotta and meat	2 shells	3	3 starch, 3 med. fat meat, 2 fat
Pasta			
With marinara sauce	1 cup	3	3 starch, 1 fat
With meat sauce	1 cup	2	2 starch, 1 veg, 1 med. fat meat, 1 fat

Food	Quantity	Carb Choices	Exchanges
Pizza			
Meat	⅛ of a 16–18 oz pizza	1	1 starch, 1 veg, 1 med. fat meat, 2 fat
Vegetarian	⅛ of a 16–18 oz pizza	2	2 starch, 1 veg, 2 fat
Ravioli			
Beef	1 cup	2	2 starch, 1 veg, 1 med. fat meat
Cheese	1 cup	2	2 starch, 1 veg, 1 med. fat meat, 2 fat
Shrimp primavera	1½ cups	0	2 veg, 3–4 lean meat, 2 fat
Spaghetti			
With meatballs	½ cup pasta with 6 small meatballs	2	2 starch, 1 veg, 2 med. fat meat
With tomato sauce	1 cup	3	3 starch, 1 veg
Tortellini	1 cup	2	2 starch, 2 veg, 2 fat
Veal cacciatore	1 cutlet with 1 cup spaghetti and ½ cup marinara sauce	3	3 starch, 3 lean meat, 1 fat
Veal marsala	1 cutlet	0	1 veg, 3 lean meat
Veal parmigiana	1 cutlet	2	2 starch, 1 veg, 3 lean meat, 1 fat

CHAPTER 14

Spicy Indian Exchanges

When many of us think of Indian food, we think "hot and spicy." But as in other cuisines, there is remarkable diversity within Indian cooking, and the level of heat differs from region to region. Foods from southern India use a lot of chiles, can be very hot, and are likely to include fish and rice. Foods from northern India are tamer, relying primarily on breads and dahls (sauces made from pureed beans or lentils). Vegetarianism is common throughout all of India, ranging from the simple exclusion of beef to the elimination of all meat, poultry, fish, and eggs.

Good Choices
Chappati, naan, or
    phulka
Brown or basmati rice
Curried chicken or fish
Curried lentils and
    chickpeas
Dahl
Chutneys
Raita
Tandoori chicken or fish
Yogurt-based sauces

Go Easy
Chicken or cheese pakoras
Dishes using cream, coconut
    oil, or milk
Fried breads such as puri,
    paratha, or puppodum
Korma dishes
Koulfi
Samosas

Sample Indian Meal

Menu	Exchanges
Puppodum, 2 small	1 starch
Tandoori murgh (barbecued chicken), 4 oz	4 lean meat, 1 fat
Alu matar (potato and pea curry), ½ cup	1 starch, 1 fat
Piaz aur tamatar ka salad (onions and tomato salad), 1 medium	1 veg
Naan, 1 small loaf	1½ starch
Basmati chawal rice, ½ cup	1 starch

Meal Total

Exchanges: 4½ starch; 1 veg; 4 lean meat; 2 fat
Calories: 700
Carbohydrate: 75 grams (41%)
Protein: 45 grams (25%)
Fat: 25 grams (34%)

Indian Food List

Food	Quantity	Carb Choices	Exchanges
Starch			
Alu mattar	1 cup	2	2 starch, 3 fat
Alu paratha	1 (6" across)	2½	2½ starch, 6 fat
Arhar, cooked	1 bowl (3" across)	1	1 starch
Arrowroot flour	2 Tbsp	1	1 starch
Barley, cooked	⅓ cup	1	1 starch
Basmati rice, cooked	½ cup	1	1 starch
Beet root	3 oz	1	1 starch
Chapati, 5–6" across	1 chapati	1	1 starch
Colocasia, cooked	¼ cup	1	1 starch
Dahl			
Uncooked	2 Tbsp	1	1 starch
Cooked	1 bowl (3" across)	1	1 starch
Dosa	1 (6" across)	1	1 starch
Idli	1 (3"across)	1	1 starch
Lentil soup	1 cup	1½	1½ starch, 1 fat
Lobia	1 small bowl	1	1 starch
Moong dal, cooked	1 medium bowl	1	1 starch
Naan	¼ large or 1 small loaf	1	1 starch
Noodles, cooked	½ cup	1	1 starch
Peas pullao	1 cup	3	3 starch
Phoa, uncooked	3 Tbsp	1	1 starch
Phulka	1 (6" across)	1	1 starch
Porridge	¾ cup	1	1 starch

Food	Quantity	Carb Choices	Exchanges
Potato	½ medium	1	1 starch
Puppodum, plain	2 small	1	1 starch
Puri	1 (5" across)	1	1 starch, 2½ fat
Rajmah	½ cup	1	1 starch
Rice, cooked	⅓ cup	1	1 starch
Rice flour, uncooked	2 Tbsp	1	1 starch
Samosa, with potato filling	1 piece	1	1 starch, 2 fat
Saag paneer	1 cup	1	1 starch, 1 fat
Upma, plain without vegetables, cooked	½ cup	1	1 starch
Whole wheat flour	3 Tbsp	1	1 starch
Fruit			
Ber (small apples)	5–8 fruits	1	1 fruit
Guava	1 medium or ½ cup	1	1 fruit
Loquat	5–6 fruits	1	1 fruit
Mango	½ medium	1	1 fruit
Papaya	½ fruit	1	1 fruit
Milk			
Carol	1 cup	1	1 milk, 1½ fat
Dahi (curds)	1 cup	1	1 milk
Khoa	2 Tbsp	1	1 milk, 1½ fat
Vegetables			
Ashgourd, cooked	½ cup	0	1 veg
Bottle gourd, cooked	1⅓ cup	0	1 veg
Bhindi	½ cup	0	1 veg
Brinjal	¾ cup	0	1 veg
Capsicum	¾ cup	0	1 veg

Food	Quantity	Carb Choices	Exchanges
Chow chow, cooked	½ cup	0	1 veg
Drumstick, cooked	½ cup	0	1 veg
Lady fingers (okra)	½ cup	0	1 veg
Lauki	¾ cup	0	1 veg
Onion chutney	¼ cup	0	1 veg
Raita	½ cup	0	1 veg
Tamata salet	½ cup	0	1 veg
Tori	¾ cup	0	1 veg
Meat/Meat Substitutes			
Chana dahl	½ cup	0	2 lean meat, 2 fat
Chicken tandoori	4 oz	0	4 lean meat, 1 fat
Lamb, chicken, fish, mutton, pork	1 oz	0	1 med. fat meat
Pakora, potato and chickpea flour	2 balls (1" across)	0	1 high fat meat, 3 fat
Paneer			
Made with skim milk	¼ cup	0	1 lean meat
Made with whole milk	¼ cup	0	1 high fat meat
Fat			
Coconut, grated, unsweetened	2 Tbsp	0	1 fat
Coconut chutney	2 Tbsp	0	1 fat
Coconut oil	1 tsp	0	1 fat
Ghee	1 tsp	0	1 fat
Oil (maize, refined, saffola, or soya)	1 tsp	0	1 fat

Food	Quantity	Carb Choices	Exchanges
Combination Dishes			
Biryani	1½ cups	3	3 starch, 1 veg, 2 lean meat, 1 fat
Kheema do pyaza	1 cup	1	1 starch, 3 med. fat meat, 2 fat
Kofta	3 balls (1½" across)	0	3 med. fat meat, 5 fat
Machli aur tamatar	3 oz	1	1 starch, 3 med. fat meat, 1 fat
Masala dosa	1 large	2	2 starch, 4 fat
Mattar paneer	½ cup	1	1 starch, 1 high fat meat, 3 fat
Murgh kari (chicken curry)	3 oz chicken	1	1 starch, 3 med. fat meat
Samosa			
Filled with lamb	1 medium (2½")	1	1 starch, 1 med. fat meat, 2 fat
Filled with peas and potatoes	1 medium (2½")	2	2 starch, 2 fat

CHAPTER 15

Exchanges for Jewish Cookery

Historically, the kosher diet has been high in fat. Many cuts of kosher meat are well-marbled with fat. Schmaltz (chicken fat) is used for flavor and sometimes as an ingredient in sandwiches. Fried dishes like blintzes (crepes) and matzo brie (fried matzo) also are popular in kosher cooking. In place of schmaltz or butter, you can use small amounts of margarine or kosher certified vegetable oil, which are pareve (neutral). Many kosher meats and poultry tend to be high in sodium, because salting is part of the koshering process.

Good Choices	*Go Easy*
Bagels	Bubke
Bean or split pea soup	Hamantaschen (purim tart)
Borscht	Hot dogs
Cabbage soup	Knockwurst
Chicken soup	Kuchen and Mandel Bread
Gefilte fish	Lekach
Kasha	Pastrami
Lox	Rugalah
Stewed fruits	Schmaltz
Turkey breast or roast beef	Teiglach

Sample Jewish Meal

Menu	Exchanges
Challah, 1 slice	1 starch
Gefilte fish, 1 oz	1 lean meat
Horseradish	free
Beet borscht, 1 cup	2 veg
Stewed chicken, 3 oz	3 high fat meat
Potato kugel, 1 cup	2 starch
Fruit compote, ½ cup	1 fruit

Meal Total

Exchanges: 3 starch; 1 fruit; 2 veg; 1 lean meat; 3 high fat meat
Calories: 700
Carbohydrate: 70 grams (40%)
Protein: 40 grams (23%)
Fat: 30 grams (38%)

Jewish Food List

Food	Quantity	Carb Choices	Exchanges
Starch			
Bagel	½ medium	1	1 starch
Bialy	½ medium	1	1 starch
Bulke	½ medium	1	1 starch
Challah (hallah)	1 slice	1	1 starch
Cream of wheat, cooked	½ cup	1	1 starch
Farfel, dry	3 Tbsp	1	1 starch
Hard roll	1 small	1	1 starch
Kasha (buckwheat groats)			
Cooked	¾ cup	2	2 starch
Dry	2 Tbsp	1	1 starch
Kichlach	3 (1" square)	1	1 starch
Lentils	⅓ cup	1	1 starch
Lokshen (noodles)	½ cup	1	1 starch
Matzo, thin	1 (1 oz)	1½	1½ starch
Matzo balls	2 balls	1	1 starch
Matzo ball soup	1 cup with 2 balls	1	1 starch, 1 fat
Matzo chips or crisps	½ cup	1½	1½ starch
Matzo crackers, 1½" square	7 crackers	1	1 starch
Mini crackers	13 crackers	1½	1½ starch
Matzo farfel, dry	¼ cup	1	1 starch
Matzo kugel	½ serving	1	1 starch, 1 fat
Matzo meal	¼ cup	1½	1½ starch
Matzo meal pancakes	1 medium	1	1 starch, 2 fat
Noodle pudding	½ cup	1½	1½ starch
Potato knish	1 (3" across)	1	1 starch, 2 fat

Food	Quantity	Carb Choices	Exchanges
Potato kugel	½ cup	1	1 starch
Potato latkes	3 latkes	1	1 starch
Potato starch (flour)	2 Tbsp	1	1 starch
Pumpernickel bread	1 slice	1	1 starch
Rye bread	1 slice	1	1 starch
Split peas, cooked	½ cup	1	1 starch
Vegetable			
Borscht	½ cup	0	1 veg, 1 fat
Sauerkraut	½ cup	0	1 veg
Sorrel (schav)	½ cup	0	1 veg
Meat/Meat Substitutes			
Beef tongue	1 oz	0	1 med. fat meat
Brisket	1 oz	0	1 med. fat meat
Caviar	1 oz	0	1 lean meat
Chicken, stewed	1 oz	0	1 high fat meat
Corned beef	1 oz	0	1 med. fat meat
Flanken	1 oz	0	1 lean meat
Gefilte fish	2 oz	0	1 lean meat
Kippered herring	1 oz	0	1 lean meat
Livers, chopped	¼ cup	0	1 med. fat meat
Lox (smoked salmon)	1 oz	0	1 lean meat
Pastrami	1 oz	0	1 high fat meat
Pickled herring	1 oz	0	1 lean meat
Pot cheese	¼ cup	0	1 lean meat
Sablefish, smoked	1 oz	0	1 med. fat meat
Salmon, pink, canned in water	1 oz	0	1 very lean meat

Food	Quantity	Carb Choices	Exchanges
Salmon, red, canned in water	1 oz	0	1 very lean meat
Sardines (canned, drained)	2 medium	0	1 lean meat
Fat			
Chicken fat (schmaltz)	1 tsp	0	1 fat
Cream cheese	1 Tbsp	0	1 fat
Grebenes	1 tsp	0	1 fat
Sour cream	2 Tbsp	0	1 fat
Light	3 Tbsp	0	1 fat
Free			
Coffee whiteners			
Nondairy liquid	1 Tbsp	0	free
Nondairy powdered	2 tsp	0	free
Horseradish	–	0	free
Pickles, dill	1½ large	0	free
Combination Dishes			
Cabbage-beet borscht	1 cup	1	1 starch, 1 fat
Cheese blintzes, frozen	8 oz entrée	2	2 starch, 2 med. fat meat, 3 fat
Chicken and dumplings	1 cup	2	2 starch, 2 med. fat meat, 1 fat
Cholent with meat	1 cup	2	2 starch, 1 veg, 2 med. fat meat; 1–2 fat
Meatless	1 cup	3	3 starch, 1–2 veg, 1–2 fat
Kreplach, meat	2 small	1	1 starch, 2 med. fat meat
Lentil soup	1 cup	2	2 starch, 1 lean meat

Food	Quantity	Carb Choices	Exchanges
Noodle pudding	½ cup	2	2 starch, 1 fat
Split pea soup	1 cup	2	2 starch, 1 lean meat
Stuffed cabbage in tomato sauce	1 large roll	1	1 starch, 1 veg, 2 med. fat meat
Tzimmes			
Carrot and apple	½ cup	2	2 starch
Sweet potato	½ cup	2	2 starch

CHAPTER 16

Exchanges for Convenience Foods

If nutrition is an important factor in our food choices, so too is convenience. The biggest problems associated with convenience foods are too much fat, too much saturated fat, and too much sodium. However, the many low-fat food products now available have made it easier to find foods that fit easily into a healthy meal plan. The Nutrition Facts panel found on every packaged food item gives you information about calories, fat, saturated fat, sodium, and other nutrients. Try to choose convenience foods that meet the nutrition guidelines in the table below.

Type of Food	Fat	Sodium
Meals and entrées	3 g or less per 100 calories	800 mg or less
Cheese	5 g or less per serving	400 mg or less per ounce
Processed meats	3 g or less per ounce	400 mg or less per ounce
Other foods	3 g or less per 15 g carbohydrate	400 mg or less per serving

Convenience Food List

Food	Quantity	Carb Choices	Exchanges
Frozen Dinners			
Dinners, 8 oz	1 dinner	2	2 starch, 1–2 med. fat meat
Dinners, 11 oz	1 dinner	2	2 starch, 1 veg, 2–3 med. fat meat, 1–2 fat
Dinners, 16 oz	1 dinner	3	3 starch, 1 veg, 3 med. fat meat, 2–3 fat
Dinners with less than 300 calories, 11 oz	1 dinner	2	2 starch, 1 veg, 1–2 lean meat
Healthy Choice® dinners, 11 oz	1 dinner	2	2 starch, 1 veg, 2 lean meat
Mexican dinners, 11 oz	1 dinner	3½	3½ starch, 1 med. fat meat, 1 fat
Oriental dinners, 9 oz	1 dinner	2	2 starch, 1 veg, 1–2 lean meat
Frozen Entrées			
Burrito	1 (5 oz)	3	3 starch, 1 med. fat meat, 1 fat
Chili with beans	1 cup	1–2	1–2 starch, 2 med. fat meat, 0–1 fat
Family-size entrées	1 cup	2	2 starch, 1–2 med. fat meat
French bread pizza	1 pizza	3	3 starch, 2 med. fat meat, 1 fat

Food	Quantity	Carb Choices	Exchanges
Hamburger Helper®	1 cup	2	2 starch, 2–3 med. fat meat, 1 fat
Hot Pockets®	1 sandwich	2½	2½ starch, 1–2 med. fat meat, 1 fat
Lasagna	1 cup	2	2 starch, 1–2 med. fat meat, 0–1 fat
Lunch Bucket®	1 bucket (8½ oz)	2	1–2 starch, 1 med. fat meat
Lunch Express® entrées	1 entrée (9 oz)	2½	2½ starch, 1–2 med. fat meat
Lunchables®, meat and cheese	1 pkg (4.5 oz)	1½	1½ starch, 3 med. fat meat, 1 fat
Macaroni and cheese	1 cup	2	2 starch, 1 med. fat meat, 1 fat
Microcup entrées	1 entrée (7.5 oz)	2	1–2 starch, 1–2 med. fat meat, 1 fat
Oriental entrées	1 entrée (13 oz)	4	3–4 starch, 1 lean meat
Oriental light entrées	1 entrée (11.25 oz)	3	2–3 starch, 1 veg, 1 lean meat
Pasta Classics®	1 entrée (12 oz)	3	3 starch, 1 veg, 2 lean meat
Pizza, 10"	¼ pizza	2	2 starch, 2 med. fat meat, 1–2 fat
Pot Pie	1 pie (7 oz)	2	2 starch, 1 veg, 1 med. fat meat, 3–4 fat

Food	Quantity	Carb Choices	Exchanges
Spaghetti dinner, canned	1 cup	2–3	2–3 starch, 1 med. fat meat, 0–1 fat
Tuna Helper®	1 cup	2	2 starch, 1–2 med. fat meat
Side Dishes			
Noodles romanoff	½ cup	1	1 starch, 1 med. fat meat, 1 fat
Potatoes, au gratin	½ cup	1½	1½ starch, 1 fat
Potato salad	½ cup	1	1 starch, 2 fat
Rice, fried with chicken and pork	1 cup	3	3 starch, 1 med. fat meat
Scalloped potatoes	½ cup	1½	1½ starch, 1 fat
Stuffing mix, microwave	½ cup	1½	1½ starch, 1–2 fat
Suddenly Salad®	¾ cup	2	2 starch, 1–2 fat
Tater tots	3 small (3 oz)	1	1 starch, 1½ fat
Twice-baked potato	½ potato (5 oz)	2	2 starch, 2 fat
Breads			
Breadsticks, average	6 breadsticks	1	1 starch
Croissants	1 medium	1½	1½ starch, 3 fat
Croissants, petite	1 small	1	1 starch, 1½ fat
Dinner rolls	1 small	1	1 starch
Muffins	1 muffin	1½	1–1½ starch, 1 fat
Light	1 muffin	1½	1½ starch
Quick bread mixes	¹⁄₁₆ loaf	1	1 starch, 1 fat

Food	Quantity	Carb Choices	Exchanges
Soups			
Bean soup	1 cup	1	1 starch, 1 very lean meat
Broth-type soup	1 cup	1	1 starch
Chunky soups	1 can (10¾ oz)	1	1 starch, 1 veg, 1 med. fat meat
Cream soups (prepared with water)	1 cup	1	1 starch, 1 fat
Cup-A-Soup*, broth-type	1 envelope (6 oz)	0	free
Cup-A-Soup*, creamy	1 envelope (6 oz)	1	1 starch
Cup O' Noodles*	1 container	2	2 starch, 3 fat
Microcup Hearty	1 container (7.5 oz)	1	1 starch, 1 lean meat
Ramen noodles	½ pkg (1½ oz)	2	2 starch, 1½ fat
Low-fat	½ pkg (1½ oz)	3	3 starch
Split pea (prepared with water)	1 cup	2	2 starch
Breakfast Items			
Egg Beaters*	½ cup	0	1 lean meat
French toast, frozen	1 slice	1	1 starch, ½ med. fat meat
Pancakes (as prepared from mix)	3 cakes (4" across)	2	2 starch, 1 fat
Microwave, 3½" across	2 cakes	1	1 starch, 1 fat
Waffles, frozen, 4½" square	1 waffle	1	1 starch, 1 fat

Food	Quantity	Carb Choices	Exchanges
Desserts			
Almost Home® cookies, all varieties	2 cookies (2 oz)	1	1 starch, 1 fat
American Collection® cookies, all varieties	1 cookie	1	1 other carb, 1 fat
Cake, fat-free	1 slice (1 oz)	1	1 other carb
Frozen dairy dessert	4 oz	1½	1½ other carb
Gingersnaps	3 cookies	1	1 other carb
Kitchen Hearth® cookies	3 cookies	1	1 other carb, 1½ fat
Lovin' Lites® cake, all varieties	1/10 cake	2½	2½ other carb
Supermoist® cake, all varieties	1/12 cake	2	2 other carb, 2 fat

CHAPTER 17

Exchanges for Smart Snacking

Each year Americans crunch their way through over twenty-five billion dollars worth of snack foods. This is not necessarily a dire statistic – although snacking often has a bad name, snacks can add both nutritional value and enjoyment to a meal plan.

Try to select snacks that provide solid nutrition and are low in fat, calories, and salt. Look for packaged snack foods that contain three grams or less fat and 400 milligrams or less sodium per serving.

Snack Food List

Food	Quantity	Carb Choices	Exchanges
Beverages			
Apple cider	½ cup	1	1 fruit
All Sport® Thirst Quencher	1 cup (8 oz)	1	1 other carb
Carnation® hot cocoa	1 pkt	1½	1½ other carb
Fat free	1 pkt	0	free
No sugar added	1 pkt	½	½ other carb

Food	Quantity	Carb Choices	Exchanges
Catawba juice	¾ cup	1	1 fruit
Chocolate milk	1 cup (8 oz)	2	2 other carb
Cocoa mix, hot, sugar free	1 pkt (6 oz)	½	½ other carb
Cranberry juice	⅓ cup	1	1 fruit
Cranberry juice, low-calorie	1 cup	1	1 fruit or 1 other carb
Fruit juice, canned	1 can (6 oz)	1½	1½ fruit
Fruit nectars (apricot, peach, pear)	⅓ cup	1	1 fruit
Gatorade®	1 cup (8 oz)	1	1 other carb
Hawaiian Punch®, low-calorie	1 cup	1	1 other carb
Powerade®	1 cup (8 oz)	1	1 other carb
Sundance® sparkling beverage	1 bottle (5 oz)	1	1 other carb
Swiss Miss® hot cocoa, fat-free	1 pkt	½	½ other carb
Light	1 pkt	1	1 other carb
No sugar added	1 pkt	1	1 other carb
Tang®	1 cup (8 oz)	1½	1½ other carb
Sugar-free	1 cup (8 oz)	0	free
Tomato juice	1½ cup	1	1 fruit
V8® juice	1 can (5.5 oz)	½	1 veg

Chips/Pretzels/Popcorn, etc.

Food	Quantity	Carb Choices	Exchanges
Bugles®, 50% less fat	1½ cups	1½	1½ starch, 1 fat
Caramel corn	½ cup (1 oz)	2	2 starch
Fat-free	¾ cup	1½	1½ starch
Caramel puff corn	¾ cup	1½	1½ starch
Cheese puffs	25 puffs (1 oz)	1	1 starch, 2 fat
Cheetos®	1 oz	1	1 starch, 2 fat

Food	Quantity	Carb Choices	Exchanges
Chex® Snack Mix	⅔ cup	1	1 starch, 1 fat
Combos®, cheddar cheese	⅓ cup	1	1 starch, 1 fat
Corn chips, all varieties	34 chips	1	1 starch, 2 fat
Cracker Jack® popcorn	½ cup	1½	1½ starch, 1 fat
Doritos® corn chips, all varieties	~34 chips (1 oz)	1	1 starch, 1 fat
Fritos® corn chips, all varieties	~34 chips (1 oz)	1	1 starch, 2 fat
Guiltless Gourmet® tortilla chips	1 oz	1½	1½ starch
Oriental rice cracker mix	½ cup	1½	1½ starch
Party mix	⅓ cup (1 oz)	1	1 starch, 1 fat
Popcorn			
Air popped	5 cups	1	1 starch
Cheese-flavored	3 cups (1 oz)	1	1 starch, 2 fat
Fat-free	3 cups (1 oz)	1	1 starch
Light	5 cups	1	1 starch, ½ fat
Microwave, with butter	5 cups	1	1 starch, 2 fat
Potato chips	12–18 chips (1 oz)	1	1 starch, 2 fat
Baked, low-fat	12–18 chips (1 oz)	1½	1½ starch, ½ fat
Fat-free	12–18 chips (1 oz)	1½	1½ starch
Reduced fat	12–18 chips (1 oz)	1	1 starch, 1 fat
Pretzels	1 oz	1½	1½ starch
Sticks, very thin	65 sticks	1	1 starch
Twists	4 twists	0	1 starch
Yogurt-covered	7 (1 oz)	1½	1½ starch, 1 fat

Food	Quantity	Carb Choices	Exchanges
Rice Cakes	2 cakes	1	1 starch
Sesame sticks	¼ cup (1 oz)	1	1 starch, 2 fat
Snack cracker mix	⅓ cup (1 oz)	1	1 starch, 1 fat
Snack mix	½ cup	1½	1½ starch, 1 fat
Reduced fat	½ cup	1½	1½ starch, 1 fat
Sun Chips®	1 oz	1	1 starch, 1 fat
Tortilla chips, fried	15–18 chips (1 oz)	1	1 starch, 1 fat
Baked	15–18 chips (1 oz)	1½	1½ starch
Trail mix	¼ cup	1	1 starch, 1 fat
Cookies			
Animal crackers	8 cookies	1	1 other carb
Archway® cookies, fat-free	1 cookie (1 oz)	1½	1½ other carb
Chips Ahoy®	3 cookies	1½	1½ other carb, 1½ fat
Reduced fat	3 cookies	1½	1½ other carb, 1 fat
Cookies, most types	1 cookie (3" across)	1	1 other carb, 1 fat
Dinosaur cookies, mini	14 cookies	1	1 other carb, ½ fat
Fig Newtons® or fig bars	2 cookies	1½	1½ other carb
Frookie®, apple cobbler	1 cookie	1	1 other carb or 1 fruit
Frookie®, animal frackers	14 cookies	1	1 other carb, 1 fat
Gingersnaps	3 cookies	1	1 other carb

Food	Quantity	Carb Choices	Exchanges
Fudge Stripe®, reduced-fat	3 cookies	1	1 other carb, 1 fat
Health Valley® jumbo fruit cookie	1 cookie	1	1 other carb
Koala yummies	13 cookies	1	1 other carb, 2 fat
Lorna Doone® shortbread	6 cookies	1	1 other carb, 1 fat
Pepperidge Farm® soft-baked reduced-fat chocolate chunk	1 cookie	1	1 other carb
Salerno® butter cookies	6 cookies	1½	1½ other carb, 1 fat
Reduced fat	6 cookies	1½	1½ other carb, 1 fat
Mini	25 cookies	1	1 other carb, 1 fat
Snackwell's® bite-size chocolate chip	13 cookies	1½	1½ other carb, ½ fat
Snackwell's® cinnamon graham snacks	20 cookies	2	2 other carb
Snackwell's® double fudge	1 cookie	1	1 other carb
Sunshine® oatmeal cookie	3 cookies	1½	1½ other carb, 1 fat
Teddy Grahams®	25 cookies	1½	1½ other carb, 1 fat
Vanilla wafers	8 cookies	1½	1½ other carb, 1 fat
Reduced fat	8 cookies	1½	1½ other carb

Food	Quantity	Carb Choices	Exchanges
Crackers			
Breadsticks, 4" long x ¼" thick	6 breadsticks	1	1 starch
Breton° wafers	6 crackers	1	1 starch, 1 fat
Reduced fat	6 crackers	1	1 starch, ½ fat
Cheese Nips°	20 crackers	1	1 starch, 1 fat
Reduced fat	22 crackers	1½	1½ starch, ½ fat
Cheez 'n Crackers°	1 package	½	½ starch, ½ med. fat meat, 1 fat
Chicken in a Biskit°	14 crackers (1 oz)	1	1 starch, 2 fat
Cracker sandwiches, reduced-fat	1 oz	1½	1½ starch, 1 fat
Garden Crisps°, vegetable	11 crackers	1	1 starch, ½ fat
Goldfish° crackers	45 crackers	1	1 starch, 1 fat
Grahams, cinnamon crisp, or chocolate	1 square (1 oz)	1½	1½ starch, 1 fat
Grahams, honey	1 square (1 oz)	1½	1½ starch, 1 fat
Harvest Crisps°, 5-Grain & Oat	12 crackers	1	1 starch, 1 fat
Hi-Ho° crackers	6 crackers	1	1 starch, 1 fat
Melba toast, long	4 slices	1	1 starch
Melba toast, rounds	8 crackers	1	1 starch
Oyster crackers	24 large or 42 small	1	1 starch
Peanut Butter 'N Cheez°	1 package	1	1 starch, ½ med. fat meat, 1 fat
Ritz°	6 crackers	1	1 starch, 1 fat
Ritz° Bits	40 crackers	1	1 starch, 1 fat

Food	Quantity	Carb Choices	Exchanges
RyKrisp®	3 crackers	1	1 starch
Snackwell's® snack crackers	32 crackers	1½	1½ starch
Snackwell's® wheat crackers	5 crackers	1	1 starch
Sociables® flavor crisps	8 crackers	1	1 starch, 1 fat
Triscuits®	6 crackers	1	1 starch, 1 fat
Vegetable Thins®	18 crackers	1½	1½ starch, 1 fat
Wasa® Bread crackers	2 slices	1	1 starch
Wheat Thins®	18 crackers	1½	1½ starch, 1 fat
Wheatables®	24 crackers (1 oz)	1	1 starch, 1 fat
Fruit Snacks			
Applesauce, natural	½ cup	1	1 fruit
Dried fruit	¼ cup (½ oz)	1	1 fruit
Fruit bar	1 bar	1	1 other carb
Fruit cup	½ cup	1	1 fruit
Fruit by the Foot®	1 roll	1	1 other carb
Fun Fruit®	1 pouch	1½	1½ other carb
Fruit juice bar, 100% juice	1 bar	1	1 other carb
Fruit Roll-Up®	1 (½ oz)	1	1 other carb
Fruit Wrinkle®	1 pouch	1½	1½ other carb
Mama Tish's® Italian Ice	½ cup	1½	1½ other carb
Nutty banana	⅔ cup	1½	1½ fruit, 3 fat
Raisins	½ oz box	1	1 fruit
Granola/Cereal Bars			
Breakfast bar	1 bar	1½	1½ other carb, 1 fat
Fudge-dipped granola bar	1 bar	1½	1½ other carb, ½ fat
Health Valley® bar	1 bar	2	2 other carb

Food	Quantity	Carb Choices	Exchanges
Nature Valley® low-fat chewy granola bar	1 bar	1½	1½ other carb
Nutri-Grain® bar	1 bar	2½	2½ other carb, ½ fat
Snackwell's® cereal bar	1 bar	2	2 other carb
Toaster pastry	1 pastry	2½	2½ other carb
Ice Cream/Frozen Snacks			
Ben & Jerry's® ice cream	½ cup	1½	1½ other carb, 3 fat
Breyers® ice cream	½ cup	1	1 other carb, 1½ fat
Fat-free	½ cup	1½	1½ other carb
Light	½ cup	1	1 other carb, 1 fat
No sugar added	½ cup	1	1 other carb, 1 fat
Breyers® low-fat frozen yogurt	½ cup	1½	1½ other carb
Colombo® nonfat frozen yogurt	½ cup	1½	1½ other carb
Dairy Queen® cone	1 small	1½	1½ other carb, 1 fat
Dannon® light frozen yogurt	½ cup	1½	1½ other carb
Dole® fruit & juice bar	1 bar	1	1 other carb
Dove® Bar, dark chocolate	1 bar	1½	1½ other carb, 3 fat
DQ® sandwich	1 sandwich	1½	1½ other carb, 1 fat

Food	Quantity	Carb Choices	Exchanges
Eskimo Pie*	1 pie	1	1 other carb, 2 fat
No sugar added	1 pie	1	1 other carb, 2 fat
Reduced fat	1 pie	1	1 other carb, 1½ fat
Fruit ice	½ cup	1	1 other carb
Fudgesicle*, no sugar added	1 bar	½	½ other carb
Haagen Dazs* ice cream	½ cup	1½	1½ other carb, 3 fat
Fat-free sorbet	½ cup	2	2 other carb
Fat-free sorbet bar	1 bar	1	1 other carb
Popsicle*	1 bar	1	1 other carb
Sugar-free	1 bar	0	free
Push-Up*	1 bar	1	1 other carb
Snackwell's* low-fat ice cream sandwich	1 sandwich	1	1 other carb
Yoplait* nonfat frozen yogurt bar	1 bar	1	1 other carb

Meat and Related Snacks

Food	Quantity	Carb Choices	Exchanges
Beef jerky	½ oz	0	1 very lean meat
Buddig* meats	1 oz	0	1 lean meat
Cheez Whiz*	2 Tbsp	0	1 high fat meat
Cottage cheese, low-fat or nonfat	¼ cup	0	1 very lean meat
Nuts	¼ cup (1 oz)	0	1 med. fat meat, 2 fat
Nut mix	¼ cup (1 oz)	½	1 med. fat meat, 2 fat
Peanut butter	1 Tbsp	0	1 high fat meat

Food	Quantity	Carb Choices	Exchanges
Pickled herring	1 oz	0	1 med. fat meat
Sardines	2 medium	0	1 lean meat
String cheese	1 oz	0	1 med. fat meat
Sunflower seeds	¼ cup (1 oz)	½	1 med. fat meat, 2 fat
Velveeta® slices or spread	1 slice or 1 oz	0	1 high fat meat
Snack Cakes/Bars/Pastries			
Hostess® cupcake, low-fat	1 (5 oz)	5	5 other carb
Kellogg's® Rice Crispy Treats®	1 bar	1	1 other carb
Muffins, fruit, fat-free, all varieties	1 small	2	1 starch, 1 fruit
Pop Tarts®, low-fat	1 tart	2½	2½ other carb
Sweet Rewards® bar	1 bar	2	2 other carb
Twinkies®, low-fat	1 cake	2	2 other carb
Soup			
Bouillon or beef broth	1 cup	0	free
Cup-A-Soup®, broth-type	6 oz	0	free
Cup-A-Soup®, cream-type	6 oz	1	1 starch
Cup-A-Soup®, Country Style	6 oz	1	1 starch
Yogurt and Pudding			
Dannon® plain lowfat yogurt	1 cup (8 oz)	1	1 milk, 1 fat
Fruit on the bottom	1 cup (8 oz)	3	1 milk, 2 other carb
Light	1 cup (8 oz)	1	1 milk
Light and crunchy	1 cup (8 oz)	2	1 milk, 1 other carb
Gelatin snack cups	1 snack (4 oz)	1	1 other carb
Sugar-free	1 snack (4 oz)	0	free

Food	Quantity	Carb Choices	Exchanges
Jell-O® sugar-free pudding	½ cup	1	1 milk or 1 other carb
Pudding cups	1 snack (4 oz)	1½	1½ other carb, 1 fat
Fat-free	1 snack (4 oz)	1½	1½ other carb

CHAPTER 18

Exchanges for Camping

Camping is becoming more popular every year, because it gives people an opportunity to get away from busy, noisy lives and to enjoy nature at its purest. Whatever type of camping you plan to do, be sure to pack enough food for the duration of the trip. It sounds obvious, but it's easy to underestimate the amount of food you'll need – people forget that increased exercise means an increased appetite. Experienced campers solve this problem by planning daily menus. Food for each day can then be packed separately and labeled with the date and time it is to be eaten. Bring slightly more food than you think you'll need, in case a pack is lost or damaged.

Sample Camping Menu

Menu	Exchanges
Breakfast	
Cooked cereal, biscuit, toast, pancakes, or French toast	4–5 starch, 3–4 fat
Fruit juice or dried fruit	1–2 fruit
Cocoa	1 other carb
Dried egg powder	1–2 meat

Morning Snack

Granola	2–3 starch, 2–3 fat

Lunch

RyKrisp®	2–3 starch
Raisins	2–3 fruit
Hard salami, cheese, or peanut butter	2–3 meat
Artificially sweetened Kool-Aid®	free

Afternoon Snack

Graham crackers, RyKrisp®, gorp, or granola bar	2–3 starch, 2–3 fat
Dried fruit, raisins	2–3 fruit
Artificially sweetened Kool-Aid®	free

Dinner

Casserole using meat	4–5 starch, 4–5 meat
Biscuits or dessert	1–2 starch, 1–2 fat
Dried vegetables	veg, as desired
Dried fruit	1–2 fruit

Evening Snack

Crackers, biscuits, or popcorn	2–3 starch, 1 fat
Cheese, peanuts, or sunflower seeds	1–2 meat
Dried fruit	1–2 fruit
Dried milk or cocoa	1 milk

Daily Total

Exchanges: 18 starch; 9 fruit; 2 milk; 1–2 veg; 10 meat; 9 fat
Calories: 3400
Carbohydrate: 440 grams (53%)
Protein: 145 grams (17%)
Fat: 115 grams (30%)

Camping Food List

Food	Quantity	Carb Choices	Exchanges
Starch			
Biscuits	1 biscuit (2")	1	1 starch, 1 fat
Cereal, cooked	½ cup	1	1 starch
Chow mein noodles	½ cup	1	1 starch, 1 fat
Corn	½ cup (1 oz dried)	1	1 starch
Cornbread	2" square	1	1 starch, 1 fat
French toast	1 slice	1	1 starch, ½ med. fat meat
Graham crackers	3 squares	1	1 starch
Hash browns, cooked	½ cup (2 oz dried)	1	1 starch, 2 fat
Hushpuppies	1 ball (2")	1	1 starch, 1 fat
Pancakes			
6" across	1 pancake	1	1 starch, 1 fat
4" across	3 pancakes	1	2 starch, 1 fat
Potatoes			
Diced	½ cup (2 oz dried)	1	1 starch
Mashed	½ cup (3 oz dried)	1	1 starch
Rice, cooked	⅓ cup	1	1 starch
RyKrisp®	3 crackers	1	1 starch
Saltine® crackers	6 crackers	1	1 starch
Soup	1 cup	1	1 starch

Food	Quantity	Carb Choices	Exchanges
Fruit			
Dried fruit	¼ cup (½ oz)	1	1 fruit
Fruit galaxie	¼ cup	1	1 fruit
Juice	½ cup	1	1 fruit
Prunes	3 medium	1	1 fruit
Raisins	2 Tbsp (½ oz)	1	1 fruit
Stewed fruit	½ cup	1	1 fruit
Milk			
Dried nonfat milk powder	⅓ cup powder	1	1 skim milk
Other Carbohydrates			
Brownie	2 x 4" piece	2	2 other carb, 2 fat
Cake, white or yellow, no icing	3" square	2	2 other carb, 2 fat
Cookies	3" across	1	1 other carb, 1 fat
Fruit bars	1 bar	1½	1½ other carb
Fruit rolls or roll-ups	1 roll (½ oz)	1	1 other carb
Gingerbread	3 x 2" piece	2	2 other carb, 2 fat
Gorp	⅓ cup	1	1 other carb, 1 fat
Granola	¼ cup	1	1 other carb, 1 fat
Granola bar	1 small bar	1	1 other carb, 1 fat
Marshmallows	2 large	1	1 other carb
Pudding	½ cup	2	2 other carb
S'mores	1 s'more	3	3 other carb, 1 fat

Food	Quantity	Carb Choices	Exchanges
Syrup, real maple	2 Tbsp	2	2 other carb
Light	2 Tbsp	1	1 other carb
Tang®	½ cup	1	1 other carb
Vanilla wafers	5 wafers	1	1 other carb
Vegetables			
Vegetables, dried	½ cup (1 oz dried)	0	1 veg
Meat			
Beef jerky	½ oz	0	1 very lean meat
Beef			
Canned	2–3 oz	0	3 lean meat
Dried	2 oz	0	3 med. fat meat
Dried, chipped	2–3 oz	0	3 lean meat
Cheese	1 oz	0	1 high fat meat
Chicken			
Canned	2–3 oz	0	3 lean meat
Dried	2 oz	0	3 lean meat
Cold cuts	1 slice (1 oz)	0	1 high fat meat
Eggs, prepared	⅓ cup	0	2 med. fat meat
Ham	1 oz	0	1 lean meat
Meat sticks	½ oz	0	1 lean meat
Meat, canned	4 oz	0	3 med. fat meat
Peanut butter	1 Tbsp	0	1 high fat meat
Peanuts	¼ cup (1 oz)	0	1 high fat meat, 1 fat
Pork chops, dried	2 oz	0	2 med. fat meat
Salami	1 slice (¼" thick or 1 oz)	0	1 high fat meat
Sardines, canned	1 oz	0	1 lean meat

Food	Quantity	Carb Choices	Exchanges
Sausage patties	2 oz	0	2 high fat meat
Shrimp, canned	1 oz	0	1 lean meat
Spam®	1 slice (3 oz)	0	3 high fat meat
Sunflower seeds	¼ cup (1 oz)	0	1 high fat meat, 1 fat
Tuna fish, canned in water	½ can (3–4 oz)	0	3 very lean meat
Combination Foods			
Baked beans and franks	1 cup	2	2 starch, 2 high fat meat
Beef stew	1 cup	1	1 starch, 2 med. fat meat, 1–2 fat
Beef stroganoff	1 cup	2	2 starch, 2 med. fat meat, 1–2 fat
Chicken à la king	1 cup	1	1 starch, 2 med. fat meat, 2 fat
Chicken and dumplings	1 cup	2	2 starch, 2 med. fat meat, 1 fat
Chili with beans	1 cup	2	2 starch, 2 lean meat
Chow mein (without noodles or rice)	2 cups	2	2 starch, 1 veg, 2 lean meat
Lasagna	1 cup	2	2 starch, 2 med. fat meat
Macaroni and cheese	1 cup	2	2 starch, 1 high fat meat
Spaghetti and meatballs	1 cup	2	2 starch, 1 veg, 2 med. fat meat
Tuna noodle casserole with peas	1 cup	2	2 starch, 1 veg, 2 med. fat meat

Resources

Nutrition

THE AMERICAN DIETETIC ASSOCIATION
216 West Jackson Boulevard, Suite 800
Chicago, IL 60606
(800) 366–1655
www.eatright.org

This organization also has a diabetes education division called the Diabetes Care and Education Dietetic Practice Group.

Diabetes

AMERICAN DIABETES ASSOCIATION
1701 North Beauregard Street
Alexandria, VA 22311
(800) 232–3472
www.diabetes.org

CANADIAN DIABETES ASSOCIATION
15 Toronto Street, Suite 800
Toronto, ON M5C 2E3 Canada
(416) 363–3373
www.diabetes.ca

AMERICAN ASSOCIATION OF DIABETES EDUCATORS

100 West Monroe, Suite 400
Chicago, IL 60603
(800) 338–3633
www.aadenet.org

INTERNATIONAL DIABETES CENTER

3800 Park Nicollet Boulevard
Minneapolis, MN 55416–2699
(888) 825-6315
www.idcdiabetes.org

JUVENILE DIABETES FOUNDATION INTERNATIONAL

120 Wall Street, 19th floor
New York, NY 10005
(212) 785-9500

NATIONAL DIABETES INFORMATION CLEARINGHOUSE

1 Information Way
Bethesda, MD 20892
(301) 654-3327
www.niddk.nih.gov

Heart Disease

THE AMERICAN HEART ASSOCIATION

7272 Greenville Avenue
Dallas, TX 75231
(800) 242–8721
www.americanheart.org

NATIONAL CHOLESTEROL EDUCATION PROGRAM INFORMATION CENTER

4733 Bethesda Avenue, Suite 530
Bethesda, MD 20814–4820
www.nhlbi.nih.gov

Camping

ALPINE AIRE

PO Box 926
Nevada City, CA 95959
> This organization makes freeze-dried camp food.

MOUNTAIN HOUSE

Oregon Freeze Dry Inc.
PO Box 1048
Albany, OR 97321
> This organization makes freeze-dried camp food.

Travel

INTERNATIONAL ASSOCIATION FOR MEDICAL ASSISTANCE TO TRAVELERS

417 Center Street
Lewiston, New York 14092
(716) 754–4883
> This organization can provide a list of doctors in foreign countries who received postgraduate training in North America or Great Britain.

INTERNATIONAL DIABETES FEDERATION

40 Washington Street
B–1050 Brussels, Belgium

This organization can provide a list of International Diabetes Federation groups that can offer assistance when you're traveling.

Books of Related Interest from IDC Publishing

FAST FOOD FACTS

Marion J. Franz, MS, RD, LD, CDE

As a definitive guide to survival in the fast-food jungle, *Fast Food Facts* shows you how to make wise selections at the top 40 fast food chains. Designed to highlight the information you need to make quick, healthy decisions. Includes meal exchanges, "smart meals" and carbohydrate choices. Also available in a pocket edition.

CONVENIENCE FOOD FACTS

Arlene Monk RD, LD, CDE and Nancy Cooper, RD, LD, CDE

Arranged for ease of comparison-shopping, *Convenience Food Facts* guides readers to low-fat choices among more than 3,000 popular brand-name products. In addition, the book lists exchange values and carbohydrate choices – information not found on food labels – for people who are using a meal planning method to lose weight or to manage a health condition such as diabetes.

THE CONVENIENCE FOODS COOKBOOK

Nancy Cooper, RD, LD, CDE

Turn brand-name foods into brand-new meals. Recipes in *The Convenience Foods Cookbook* transform packaged goods into time-saving dishes. Healthy dishes go from package to plate in just under 20 minutes. Nutrition information, food exchanges, and carbohydrate choices included for all recipes.

These publications are available at your local bookstore or by calling 1-888-637-2675.

Visit our website at www.idcpublishing.com.